AROMATHERAPY CERTIFICATION PROGRAM WORKBOOK

REBECCA PARK TOTILO

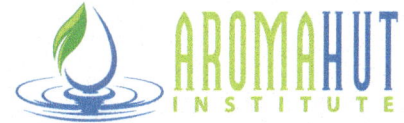

Copyright

This course has been designed to educate laypersons and health practitioners on the safe use of essential oils and clinical aromatherapy. It is offered with the understanding that Rebecca at the Well Foundation and/or Aroma Hut Institute or Rebecca Totilo shall not have any liability or reprehensibility for any injury caused directly or indirectly by the information contained in this course. Every effort has been taken to provide accurate information, however, none of the information in this course should be considered as medical advice or treatment. Please seek medical advice and recommendations for appropriate healthcare from a qualified medical health care provider if needed.

Copyright © 2015 Rebecca Park Totilo
All Rights Reserved.

This course may not be reproduced or transmitted in any form or by any means, electronic, mechanical, including photocopying, recording, or by any information storage or retrieval system without written permission from Rebecca at the Well Foundation.

Rebecca at the Well Foundation
P.O. Box 60044
Saint Petersburg, Florida 33784

Rebecca at the Well Foundation http://RebeccaAtTheWell.org
Aroma Hut Institute http://AromaHut.org

ISBN 978-0-9898280-8-6

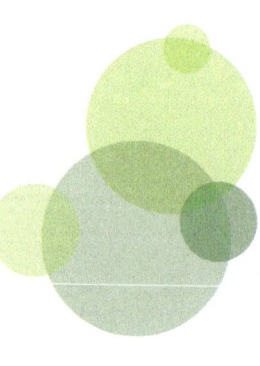

CONTENTS

Aromatic Blend Forms	1
Therapeutic Blend Forms	13
Recipe Reports	41
Aromatherapy Client Intake Forms	69
Apothecary Notes	191
Essential Oil Datasheet Forms	223

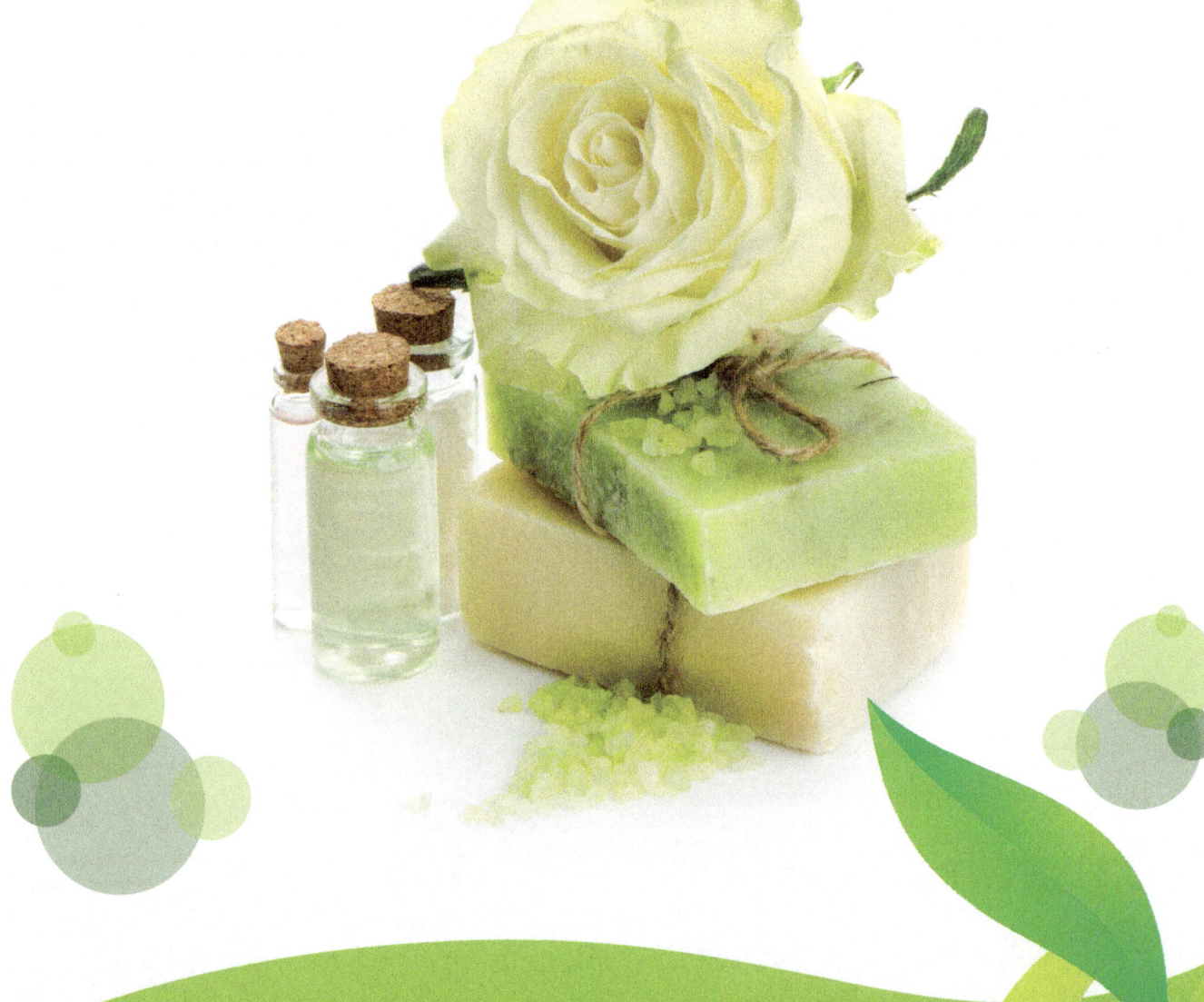

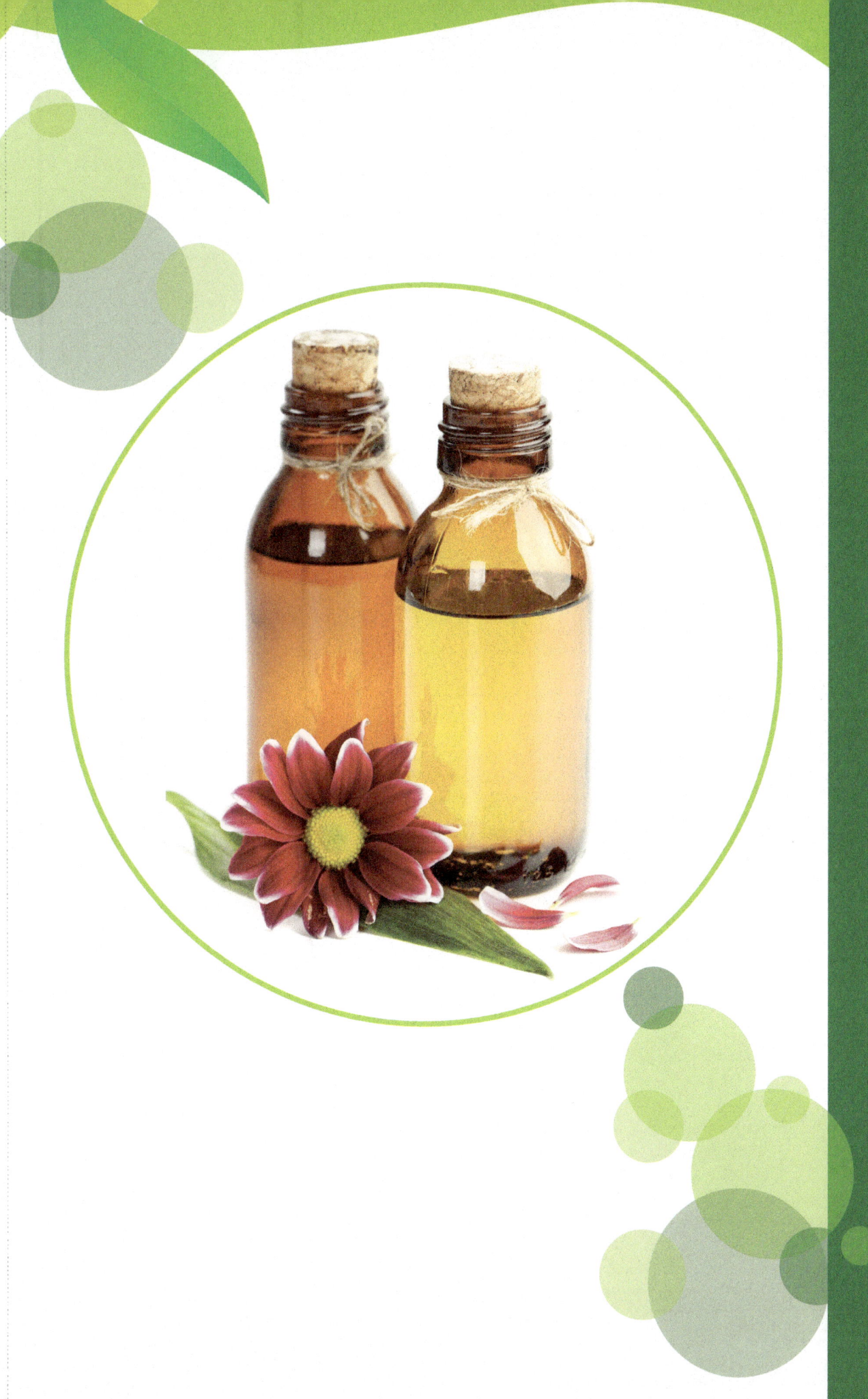

AROMATIC BLEND FORMS

ACP-1 ACTIVITY: AROMATIC BLEND FORM

Use This Form to Record Your Aromatic Essential Oil Blend.

Name of Blend: _____   Date: _____ / _____ / _____

Purpose of Blend: _____
_____
_____
_____
_____

Carriers Used: _____
_____
_____
_____
_____

Note: Essential Oils: Drops:

ACP-1 ACTIVITY: AROMATIC BLEND FORM

ACP-1 ACTIVITY: AROMATIC BLEND FORM

Use This Form to Record Your Aromatic Essential Oil Blend.

Name of Blend: ☐   Date: _____ / _____ / _____

Purpose of Blend: _____
_____
_____
_____
_____

Carriers Used: _____
_____
_____
_____
_____

Note:	Essential Oils:	Drops:

ACP-1 ACTIVITY: AROMATIC BLEND FORM

Use This Form to Record Your Aromatic Essential Oil Blend.

Name of Blend: _____   Date: _____ / _____ / _____

Purpose of Blend: _____
_____
_____
_____
_____

Carriers Used: _____
_____
_____
_____
_____

Note:	Essential Oils:	Drops:

ACP-1 ACTIVITY: AROMATIC BLEND FORM

ACP-1 ACTIVITY: AROMATIC BLEND FORM

Use This Form to Record Your Aromatic Essential Oil Blend.

Name of Blend: _____ Date: _____ / _____ / _____

Purpose of Blend: _____
_____
_____
_____
_____

Carriers Used: _____
_____
_____
_____
_____

Note:	Essential Oils:	Drops:

ACP-1 ACTIVITY: AROMATIC BLEND FORM

Use This Form to Record Your Aromatic Essential Oil Blend.

Name of Blend: _____   Date: ____ / ____ / ____

Purpose of Blend: _____
_____
_____
_____
_____

Carriers Used: _____
_____
_____
_____
_____

Note:	Essential Oils:	Drops:

ACP-1 ACTIVITY: AROMATIC BLEND FORM

Use This Form to Record Your Aromatic Essential Oil Blend.

Name of Blend: _____   Date: _____ / _____ / _____

Purpose of Blend: _____
_____
_____
_____
_____

Carriers Used: _____
_____
_____
_____
_____

Note:	Essential Oils:	Drops:

ACP-1 ACTIVITY: AROMATIC BLEND FORM

Use This Form to Record Your Aromatic Essential Oil Blend.

Name of Blend: _____   Date: _____ / _____ / _____

Purpose of Blend: _____
_____
_____
_____
_____

Carriers Used: _____
_____
_____
_____
_____

Note: Essential Oils: Drops:

ACP-1 ACTIVITY: AROMATIC BLEND FORM

ACP-1 ACTIVITY: AROMATIC BLEND FORM

Use This Form to Record Your Aromatic Essential Oil Blend.

Name of Blend: _____ Date: _____ / _____ / _____

Purpose of Blend: _____
_____
_____
_____
_____

Carriers Used: _____
_____
_____
_____
_____

Note:	Essential Oils:	Drops:

ACP-1 ACTIVITY: AROMATIC BLEND FORM

Use This Form to Record Your Aromatic Essential Oil Blend.

Name of Blend: _____ Date: _____ / _____ / _____

Purpose of Blend: _____
_____
_____
_____
_____

Carriers Used: _____
_____
_____
_____
_____

Note:	Essential Oils:	Drops:

ACP-1 ACTIVITY: AROMATIC BLEND FORM

ACP-1 ACTIVITY: AROMATIC BLEND FORM

Use This Form to Record Your Aromatic Essential Oil Blend.

Name of Blend: _____   Date: _____ / _____ / _____

Purpose of Blend: _____
_____
_____
_____
_____

Carriers Used: _____
_____
_____
_____
_____

Note:	Essential Oils:	Drops:

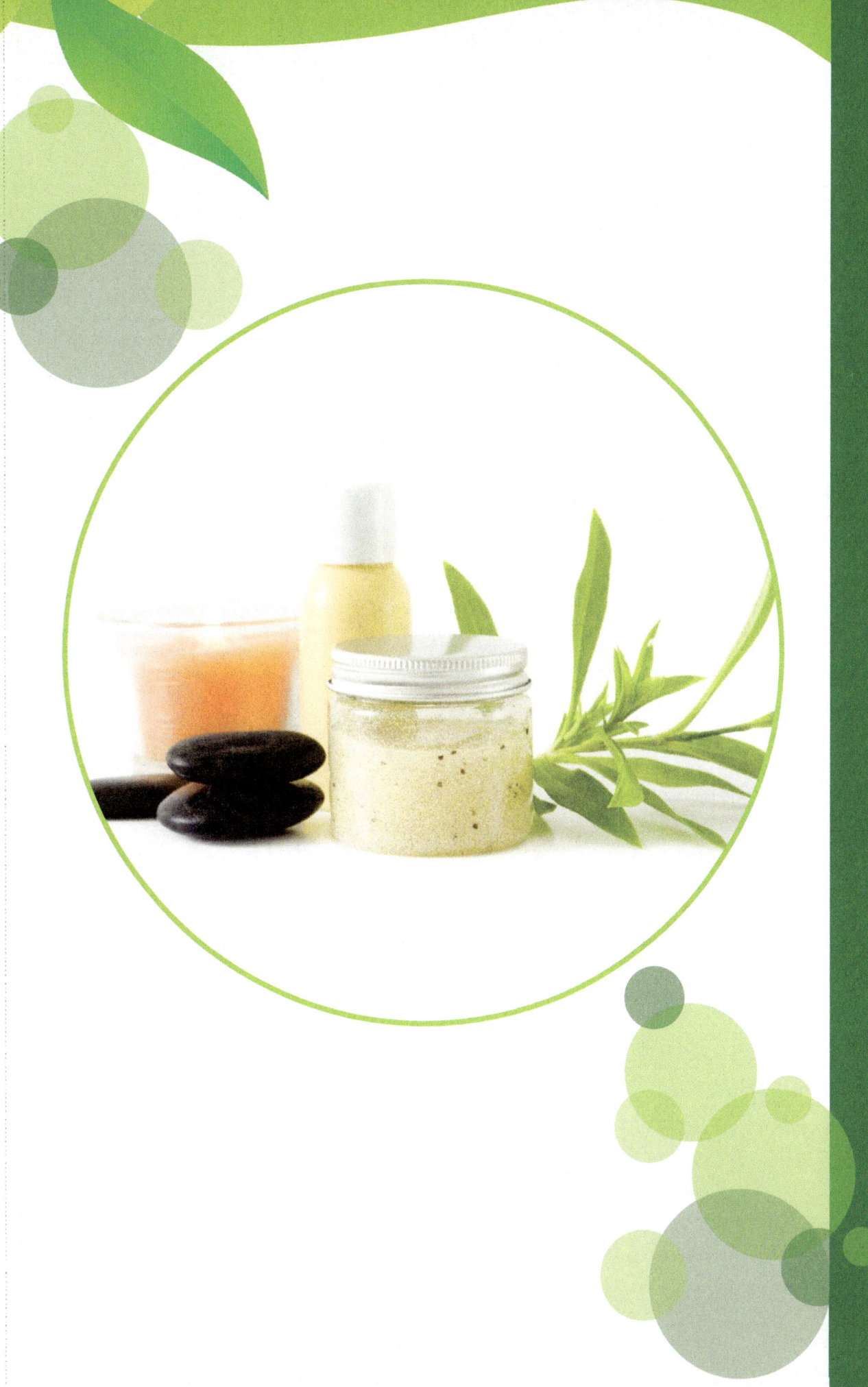

THERAPEUTIC BLEND FORMS

ACP-1 ACTIVITY: THERAPEUTIC BLEND FORM

Use This Form to Record Your Therapeutic Essential Oil Blend.

Name of Blend: _____   Date: _____ / _____ / _____

Purpose of Blend: _____
_____
_____
_____
_____

Carriers Used: _____
_____
_____
_____
_____

Note: Essential Oils: Drops:

ACP-1 ACTIVITY: THERAPEUTIC BLEND FORM

Use This Form to Record Your Therapeutic Essential Oil Blend.

Name of Blend: _____ Date: _____ / _____ / _____

Purpose of Blend: _____
_____
_____
_____
_____

Carriers Used: _____
_____
_____
_____
_____

Note:	Essential Oils:	Drops:

ACP-1 ACTIVITY: THERAPEUTIC BLEND FORM

Use This Form to Record Your Therapeutic Essential Oil Blend.

Name of Blend: _____   Date: _____ / _____ / _____

Purpose of Blend: _____
_____
_____
_____
_____

Carriers Used: _____
_____
_____
_____
_____

Note:	Essential Oils:	Drops:

ACP-1 ACTIVITY: THERAPEUTIC BLEND FORM

ACP-1 ACTIVITY: THERAPEUTIC BLEND FORM

Use This Form to Record Your Therapeutic Essential Oil Blend.

Name of Blend: _____   Date: _____ / _____ / _____

Purpose of Blend: _____
_____
_____
_____
_____

Carriers Used: _____
_____
_____
_____
_____

Note:	Essential Oils:	Drops:

ACP-1 ACTIVITY: THERAPEUTIC BLEND FORM

Use This Form to Record Your Therapeutic Essential Oil Blend.

Name of Blend: _____   Date: _____ / _____ / _____

Purpose of Blend: _____
_____
_____
_____
_____

Carriers Used: _____
_____
_____
_____
_____

Note:	Essential Oils:	Drops:

ACP-1 ACTIVITY: THERAPEUTIC BLEND FORM

ACP-1 ACTIVITY: THERAPEUTIC BLEND FORM

Use This Form to Record Your Therapeutic Essential Oil Blend.

Name of Blend: _____   Date: _____ / _____ / _____

Purpose of Blend: _____
_____
_____
_____
_____

Carriers Used: _____
_____
_____
_____
_____

Note:	Essential Oils:	Drops:

ACP-1 ACTIVITY: THERAPEUTIC BLEND FORM

Use This Form to Record Your Therapeutic Essential Oil Blend.

Name of Blend: _____   Date: _____ / _____ / _____

Purpose of Blend: _____
_____
_____
_____
_____

Carriers Used: _____
_____
_____
_____
_____

Note:	Essential Oils:	Drops:

ACP-1 ACTIVITY: THERAPEUTIC BLEND FORM

ACP-1 ACTIVITY: THERAPEUTIC BLEND FORM

Use This Form to Record Your Therapeutic Essential Oil Blend.

Name of Blend: _____   Date: _____ / _____ / _____

Purpose of Blend: _____
_____
_____
_____
_____

Carriers Used: _____
_____
_____
_____
_____

Note:	Essential Oils:	Drops:

ACP-1 ACTIVITY: THERAPEUTIC BLEND FORM

Use This Form to Record Your Therapeutic Essential Oil Blend.

Name of Blend: _____   Date: _____ / _____ / _____

Purpose of Blend: _____
_____
_____
_____
_____

Carriers Used: _____
_____
_____
_____
_____

Note:	Essential Oils:	Drops:

ACP-1 ACTIVITY: THERAPEUTIC BLEND FORM

23

ACP-1 ACTIVITY: THERAPEUTIC BLEND FORM

Use This Form to Record Your Therapeutic Essential Oil Blend.

Name of Blend: _____   Date: _____ / _____ / _____

Purpose of Blend: _____
_____
_____
_____
_____

Carriers Used: _____
_____
_____
_____
_____

Note:	Essential Oils:	Drops:

ACP-1 ACTIVITY: THERAPEUTIC BLEND FORM

Use This Form to Record Your Therapeutic Essential Oil Blend.

Name of Blend: _____   Date: _____ / _____ / _____

Purpose of Blend: _____
_____
_____
_____
_____

Carriers Used: _____
_____
_____
_____
_____

Note:	Essential Oils:	Drops:

ACP-1 ACTIVITY: THERAPEUTIC BLEND FORM

Use This Form to Record Your Therapeutic Essential Oil Blend.

Name of Blend: [   ]   Date: ____ / ____ / ____

Purpose of Blend: _____
_____
_____
_____
_____

Carriers Used: _____
_____
_____
_____
_____

Note:	Essential Oils:	Drops:

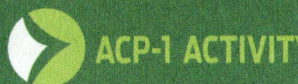

ACP-1 ACTIVITY: THERAPEUTIC BLEND FORM

Use This Form to Record Your Therapeutic Essential Oil Blend.

Name of Blend: _____   Date: _____ / _____ / _____

Purpose of Blend: _____
_____
_____
_____
_____

Carriers Used: _____
_____
_____
_____
_____

Note:	Essential Oils:	Drops:

ACP-1 ACTIVITY: **THERAPEUTIC BLEND FORM**

ACP-1 ACTIVITY: THERAPEUTIC BLEND FORM

Use This Form to Record Your Therapeutic Essential Oil Blend.

Name of Blend: _____ Date: _____ / _____ / _____

Purpose of Blend: _____
_____
_____
_____
_____

Carriers Used: _____
_____
_____
_____
_____

Note: Essential Oils: Drops:

ACP-1 ACTIVITY: THERAPEUTIC BLEND FORM

Use This Form to Record Your Therapeutic Essential Oil Blend.

Name of Blend: _____ Date: _____ / _____ / _____

Purpose of Blend: _____
_____
_____
_____
_____

Carriers Used: _____
_____
_____
_____
_____

Note:	Essential Oils:	Drops:

ACP-1 ACTIVITY: THERAPEUTIC BLEND FORM

29

ACP-1 ACTIVITY: THERAPEUTIC BLEND FORM

Use This Form to Record Your Therapeutic Essential Oil Blend.

Name of Blend: _____ Date: _____ / _____ / _____

Purpose of Blend: _____
_____
_____
_____
_____

Carriers Used: _____
_____
_____
_____
_____

Note:	Essential Oils:	Drops:

ACP-1 ACTIVITY: THERAPEUTIC BLEND FORM

Use This Form to Record Your Therapeutic Essential Oil Blend.

Name of Blend: [   ]   Date: _____ / _____ / _____

Purpose of Blend: _____
_____
_____
_____
_____

Carriers Used: _____
_____
_____
_____
_____

Note:	Essential Oils:	Drops:

ACP-1 ACTIVITY: THERAPEUTIC BLEND FORM

ACP-1 ACTIVITY: THERAPEUTIC BLEND FORM

Use This Form to Record Your Therapeutic Essential Oil Blend.

Name of Blend: _____   Date: _____ / _____ / _____

Purpose of Blend: _____
_____
_____
_____
_____

Carriers Used: _____
_____
_____
_____
_____

Note:	Essential Oils:	Drops:

ACP-1 ACTIVITY: THERAPEUTIC BLEND FORM

Use This Form to Record Your Therapeutic Essential Oil Blend.

Name of Blend: _____   Date: _____ / _____ / _____

Purpose of Blend: _____
_____
_____
_____
_____

Carriers Used: _____
_____
_____
_____
_____

Note:	Essential Oils:	Drops:

ACP-1 ACTIVITY: THERAPEUTIC BLEND FORM

ACP-1 ACTIVITY: THERAPEUTIC BLEND FORM

Use This Form to Record Your Therapeutic Essential Oil Blend.

Name of Blend: _____   Date: _____ / _____ / _____

Purpose of Blend: _____
_____
_____
_____
_____

Carriers Used: _____
_____
_____
_____
_____

Note:	Essential Oils:	Drops:

ACP-1 ACTIVITY: THERAPEUTIC BLEND FORM

Use This Form to Record Your Therapeutic Essential Oil Blend.

Name of Blend: _____ Date: ____ / ____ / ____

Purpose of Blend: _____
_____
_____
_____
_____

Carriers Used: _____
_____
_____
_____
_____

Note:	Essential Oils:	Drops:

ACP-1 ACTIVITY: THERAPEUTIC BLEND FORM

ACP-1 ACTIVITY: THERAPEUTIC BLEND FORM

Use This Form to Record Your Therapeutic Essential Oil Blend.

Name of Blend: _____ Date: _____ / _____ / _____

Purpose of Blend: _____
_____
_____
_____
_____

Carriers Used: _____
_____
_____
_____
_____

Note:	Essential Oils:	Drops:

ACP-1 ACTIVITY: THERAPEUTIC BLEND FORM

Use This Form to Record Your Therapeutic Essential Oil Blend.

Name of Blend: Date: ____ / ____ / ____

Purpose of Blend: _____
_____
_____
_____
_____

Carriers Used: _____
_____
_____
_____
_____

Note:	Essential Oils:	Drops:

ACP-1 ACTIVITY: THERAPEUTIC BLEND FORM

ACP-1 ACTIVITY: THERAPEUTIC BLEND FORM

Use This Form to Record Your Therapeutic Essential Oil Blend.

Name of Blend: _____ Date: _____ / _____ / _____

Purpose of Blend: _____
_____
_____
_____
_____

Carriers Used: _____
_____
_____
_____
_____

Note:	Essential Oils:	Drops:

ACP-1 ACTIVITY: THERAPEUTIC BLEND FORM

Use This Form to Record Your Therapeutic Essential Oil Blend.

Name of Blend: _____ Date: _____ / _____ / _____

Purpose of Blend: _____
_____
_____
_____
_____

Carriers Used: _____
_____
_____
_____
_____

Note:	Essential Oils:	Drops:

ACP-1 ACTIVITY: THERAPEUTIC BLEND FORM

Use This Form to Record Your Therapeutic Essential Oil Blend.

Name of Blend: _____   Date: _____ / _____ / _____

Purpose of Blend: _____
_____
_____
_____
_____

Carriers Used: _____
_____
_____
_____
_____

Note:	Essential Oils:	Drops:

RECIPE REPORTS

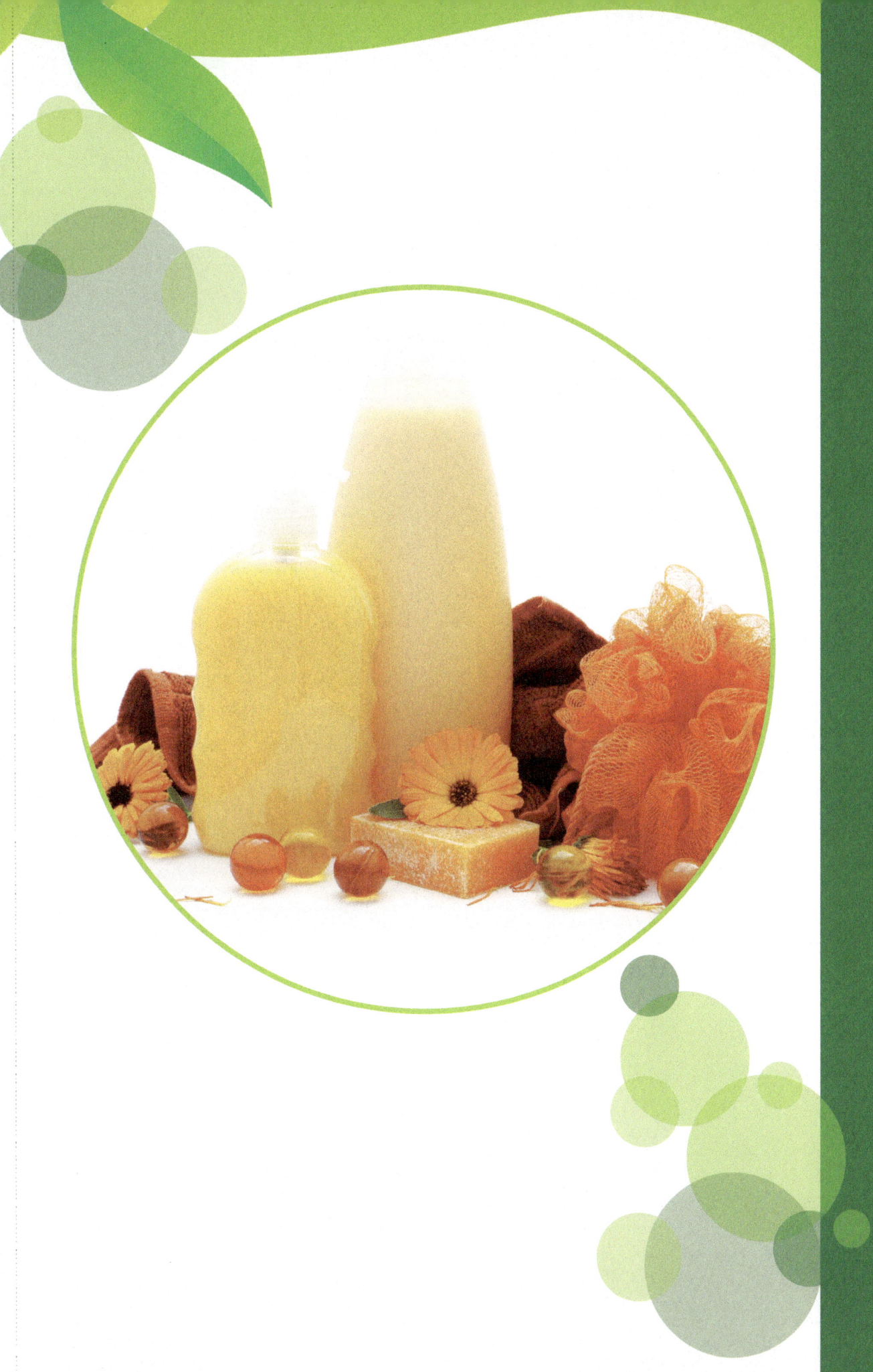

RECIPE REPORT

Please use this form to share your experience when trying out a new recipe for creating your product. Feel free to expand on any question with details.

Recipe You Tried: _____

Name Given to Your Product: _____

Purpose (circle one): Aromatic or Therapeutic

Product Description: _____

_____

_____

Time to Prepare: _____

Instructions For Use: _____

_____

_____

_____

How Often Was it Used? _____

Did the Product Work?   Yes ☐   No ☐

FINAL RESULTS
What would you change or do differently next time?

_____

_____

_____

_____

RECIPE REPORT

*Please use this form to share your experience when trying
out a new recipe for creating your product.
Feel free to expand on any question with details.*

Recipe You Tried: _____

Name Given to Your Product: _____

Purpose (circle one): Aromatic or Therapeutic

Product Description: _____
_____
_____

Time to Prepare: _____

Instructions For Use: _____
_____
_____
_____

How Often Was it Used? _____

Did the Product Work?   Yes ☐   No ☐

FINAL RESULTS
What would you change or do differently next time?

_____
_____
_____
_____

RECIPE REPORT

Please use this form to share your experience when trying out a new recipe for creating your product. Feel free to expand on any question with details.

Recipe You Tried: _____

Name Given to Your Product: _____

Purpose (circle one): Aromatic or Therapeutic

Product Description: _____
_____
_____

Time to Prepare: _____

Instructions For Use: _____
_____
_____
_____

How Often Was it Used? _____

Did the Product Work?   Yes ☐   No ☐

FINAL RESULTS
What would you change or do differently next time?

_____
_____
_____
_____

RECIPE REPORT

*Please use this form to share your experience when trying
out a new recipe for creating your product.
Feel free to expand on any question with details.*

Recipe You Tried: _____

Name Given to Your Product: _____

Purpose (circle one): Aromatic or Therapeutic

Product Description: _____
_____
_____

Time to Prepare: _____

Instructions For Use: _____
_____
_____
_____

How Often Was it Used? _____

Did the Product Work?   Yes ☐   No ☐

FINAL RESULTS
What would you change or do differently next time?

_____
_____
_____
_____

RECIPE REPORT

Please use this form to share your experience when trying out a new recipe for creating your product. Feel free to expand on any question with details.

Recipe You Tried: _____

Name Given to Your Product: _____

Purpose (circle one): Aromatic or Therapeutic

Product Description: _____
_____
_____

Time to Prepare: _____

Instructions For Use: _____
_____
_____
_____

How Often Was it Used? _____

Did the Product Work?   Yes ☐   No ☐

FINAL RESULTS
What would you change or do differently next time?

_____
_____
_____
_____

RECIPE REPORT

Please use this form to share your experience when trying out a new recipe for creating your product. Feel free to expand on any question with details.

Recipe You Tried: _____

Name Given to Your Product: _____

Purpose (circle one): Aromatic or Therapeutic

Product Description: _____
_____
_____

Time to Prepare: _____

Instructions For Use: _____
_____
_____
_____

How Often Was it Used? _____

Did the Product Work?   Yes ☐   No ☐

FINAL RESULTS
What would you change or do differently next time?

_____
_____
_____
_____

RECIPE REPORT

Please use this form to share your experience when trying out a new recipe for creating your product. Feel free to expand on any question with details.

Recipe You Tried: _____

Name Given to Your Product: _____

Purpose (circle one): Aromatic or Therapeutic

Product Description: _____
_____
_____

Time to Prepare: _____

Instructions For Use: _____
_____
_____
_____

How Often Was it Used? _____

Did the Product Work?   Yes [ ]   No [ ]

FINAL RESULTS
What would you change or do differently next time?

_____
_____
_____
_____

RECIPE REPORT

Please use this form to share your experience when trying out a new recipe for creating your product. Feel free to expand on any question with details.

Recipe You Tried: _____

Name Given to Your Product: _____

Purpose (circle one): Aromatic or Therapeutic

Product Description: _____
_____
_____

Time to Prepare: _____

Instructions For Use: _____
_____
_____
_____

How Often Was it Used? _____

Did the Product Work?   Yes ☐   No ☐

FINAL RESULTS
What would you change or do differently next time?

_____
_____
_____
_____
_____

RECIPE REPORT

Please use this form to share your experience when trying out a new recipe for creating your product. Feel free to expand on any question with details.

Recipe You Tried: _____

Name Given to Your Product: _____

Purpose (circle one): Aromatic or Therapeutic

Product Description: _____
_____
_____

Time to Prepare: _____

Instructions For Use: _____
_____
_____
_____

How Often Was it Used? _____

Did the Product Work?   Yes [ ]   No [ ]

FINAL RESULTS
What would you change or do differently next time?

_____
_____
_____
_____

RECIPE REPORT

*Please use this form to share your experience when trying
out a new recipe for creating your product.
Feel free to expand on any question with details.*

Recipe You Tried: _____

Name Given to Your Product: _____

Purpose (circle one): Aromatic or Therapeutic

Product Description: _____
_____
_____

Time to Prepare: _____

Instructions For Use: _____
_____
_____
_____

How Often Was it Used? _____

Did the Product Work?   Yes ☐   No ☐

FINAL RESULTS
What would you change or do differently next time?

_____
_____
_____
_____

RECIPE REPORT

*Please use this form to share your experience when trying
out a new recipe for creating your product.
Feel free to expand on any question with details.*

Recipe You Tried: _____

Name Given to Your Product: _____

Purpose (circle one): Aromatic or Therapeutic

Product Description: _____
_____
_____

Time to Prepare: _____

Instructions For Use: _____
_____
_____
_____

How Often Was it Used? _____

Did the Product Work?   Yes ☐   No ☐

FINAL RESULTS
What would you change or do differently next time?

_____
_____
_____
_____
_____

RECIPE REPORT

Please use this form to share your experience when trying out a new recipe for creating your product. Feel free to expand on any question with details.

Recipe You Tried: _____

Name Given to Your Product: _____

Purpose (circle one): Aromatic or Therapeutic

Product Description: _____
_____
_____

Time to Prepare: _____

Instructions For Use: _____
_____
_____
_____

How Often Was it Used? _____

Did the Product Work?   Yes ☐   No ☐

FINAL RESULTS
What would you change or do differently next time?

_____
_____
_____
_____

RECIPE REPORT

*Please use this form to share your experience when trying
out a new recipe for creating your product.
Feel free to expand on any question with details.*

Recipe You Tried: _____

Name Given to Your Product: _____

Purpose (circle one): Aromatic or Therapeutic

Product Description: _____
_____
_____

Time to Prepare: _____

Instructions For Use: _____
_____
_____
_____

How Often Was it Used? _____

Did the Product Work?   Yes ☐   No ☐

FINAL RESULTS
What would you change or do differently next time?

_____
_____
_____
_____
_____

RECIPE REPORT

*Please use this form to share your experience when trying
out a new recipe for creating your product.
Feel free to expand on any question with details.*

Recipe You Tried: _____

Name Given to Your Product: _____

Purpose (circle one): Aromatic or Therapeutic

Product Description: _____
_____
_____

Time to Prepare: _____

Instructions For Use: _____
_____
_____
_____

How Often Was it Used? _____

Did the Product Work?   Yes ☐   No ☐

FINAL RESULTS
What would you change or do differently next time?

_____
_____
_____
_____

RECIPE REPORT

Please use this form to share your experience when trying out a new recipe for creating your product. Feel free to expand on any question with details.

Recipe You Tried: _____

Name Given to Your Product: _____

Purpose (circle one): Aromatic or Therapeutic

Product Description: _____
_____
_____

Time to Prepare: _____

Instructions For Use: _____
_____
_____
_____

How Often Was it Used? _____

Did the Product Work? Yes ☐   No ☐

FINAL RESULTS
What would you change or do differently next time?

_____
_____
_____
_____

RECIPE REPORT

Please use this form to share your experience when trying out a new recipe for creating your product. Feel free to expand on any question with details.

Recipe You Tried: _____

Name Given to Your Product: _____

Purpose (circle one): Aromatic or Therapeutic

Product Description: _____
_____
_____

Time to Prepare: _____

Instructions For Use: _____
_____
_____
_____

How Often Was it Used? _____

Did the Product Work?   Yes [ ]   No [ ]

FINAL RESULTS
What would you change or do differently next time?

_____
_____
_____
_____

RECIPE REPORT

*Please use this form to share your experience when trying
out a new recipe for creating your product.
Feel free to expand on any question with details.*

Recipe You Tried: _____

Name Given to Your Product: _____

Purpose (circle one): Aromatic or Therapeutic

Product Description: _____
_____
_____

Time to Prepare: _____

Instructions For Use: _____
_____
_____
_____

How Often Was it Used? _____

Did the Product Work?   Yes ☐   No ☐

FINAL RESULTS
What would you change or do differently next time?

_____
_____
_____
_____

RECIPE REPORT

Please use this form to share your experience when trying out a new recipe for creating your product. Feel free to expand on any question with details.

Recipe You Tried: _____

Name Given to Your Product: _____

Purpose (circle one): Aromatic or Therapeutic

Product Description: _____
_____
_____

Time to Prepare: _____

Instructions For Use: _____
_____
_____
_____

How Often Was it Used? _____

Did the Product Work?   Yes ☐   No ☐

FINAL RESULTS
What would you change or do differently next time?

_____
_____
_____
_____

RECIPE REPORT

Please use this form to share your experience when trying out a new recipe for creating your product. Feel free to expand on any question with details.

Recipe You Tried: _____

Name Given to Your Product: _____

Purpose (circle one): Aromatic or Therapeutic

Product Description: _____
_____
_____

Time to Prepare: _____

Instructions For Use: _____
_____
_____
_____

How Often Was it Used? _____

Did the Product Work?   Yes ☐   No ☐

FINAL RESULTS
What would you change or do differently next time?

_____
_____
_____
_____

RECIPE REPORT

*Please use this form to share your experience when trying
out a new recipe for creating your product.
Feel free to expand on any question with details.*

Recipe You Tried: _____

Name Given to Your Product: _____

Purpose (circle one): Aromatic or Therapeutic

Product Description: _____
_____
_____

Time to Prepare: _____

Instructions For Use: _____
_____
_____
_____

How Often Was it Used? _____

Did the Product Work?   Yes ☐   No ☐

FINAL RESULTS
What would you change or do differently next time?

_____
_____
_____
_____

RECIPE REPORT

Please use this form to share your experience when trying out a new recipe for creating your product. Feel free to expand on any question with details.

Recipe You Tried: _____

Name Given to Your Product: _____

Purpose (circle one): Aromatic or Therapeutic

Product Description: _____
_____
_____

Time to Prepare: _____

Instructions For Use: _____
_____
_____
_____

How Often Was it Used? _____

Did the Product Work?   Yes ☐   No ☐

FINAL RESULTS
What would you change or do differently next time?

_____
_____
_____
_____

RECIPE REPORT

Please use this form to share your experience when trying out a new recipe for creating your product. Feel free to expand on any question with details.

Recipe You Tried: _____

Name Given to Your Product: _____

Purpose (circle one): Aromatic or Therapeutic

Product Description: _____
_____
_____

Time to Prepare: _____

Instructions For Use: _____
_____
_____
_____

How Often Was it Used? _____

Did the Product Work?   Yes [ ]   No [ ]

FINAL RESULTS
What would you change or do differently next time?

_____
_____
_____
_____

RECIPE REPORT

Please use this form to share your experience when trying out a new recipe for creating your product. Feel free to expand on any question with details.

Recipe You Tried: _____

Name Given to Your Product: _____

Purpose (circle one): Aromatic or Therapeutic

Product Description: _____
_____
_____

Time to Prepare: _____

Instructions For Use: _____
_____
_____
_____

How Often Was it Used? _____

Did the Product Work?   Yes ☐   No ☐

FINAL RESULTS
What would you change or do differently next time?

_____
_____
_____
_____

RECIPE REPORT

*Please use this form to share your experience when trying
out a new recipe for creating your product.
Feel free to expand on any question with details.*

Recipe You Tried: _____

Name Given to Your Product: _____

Purpose (circle one): Aromatic or Therapeutic

Product Description: _____
_____
_____

Time to Prepare: _____

Instructions For Use: _____
_____
_____
_____

How Often Was it Used? _____

Did the Product Work?   Yes ☐   No ☐

FINAL RESULTS
What would you change or do differently next time?

_____
_____
_____
_____
_____

RECIPE REPORT

Please use this form to share your experience when trying out a new recipe for creating your product. Feel free to expand on any question with details.

Recipe You Tried: _____

Name Given to Your Product: _____

Purpose (circle one): Aromatic or Therapeutic

Product Description: _____
_____
_____

Time to Prepare: _____

Instructions For Use: _____
_____
_____
_____

How Often Was it Used? _____

Did the Product Work?   Yes ☐   No ☐

FINAL RESULTS
What would you change or do differently next time?

_____
_____
_____
_____
_____

RECIPE REPORT

Please use this form to share your experience when trying out a new recipe for creating your product. Feel free to expand on any question with details.

Recipe You Tried: _____

Name Given to Your Product: _____

Purpose (circle one): Aromatic or Therapeutic

Product Description: _____
_____
_____

Time to Prepare: _____

Instructions For Use: _____
_____
_____
_____

How Often Was it Used? _____

Did the Product Work?   Yes ☐   No ☐

FINAL RESULTS
What would you change or do differently next time?

_____
_____
_____
_____

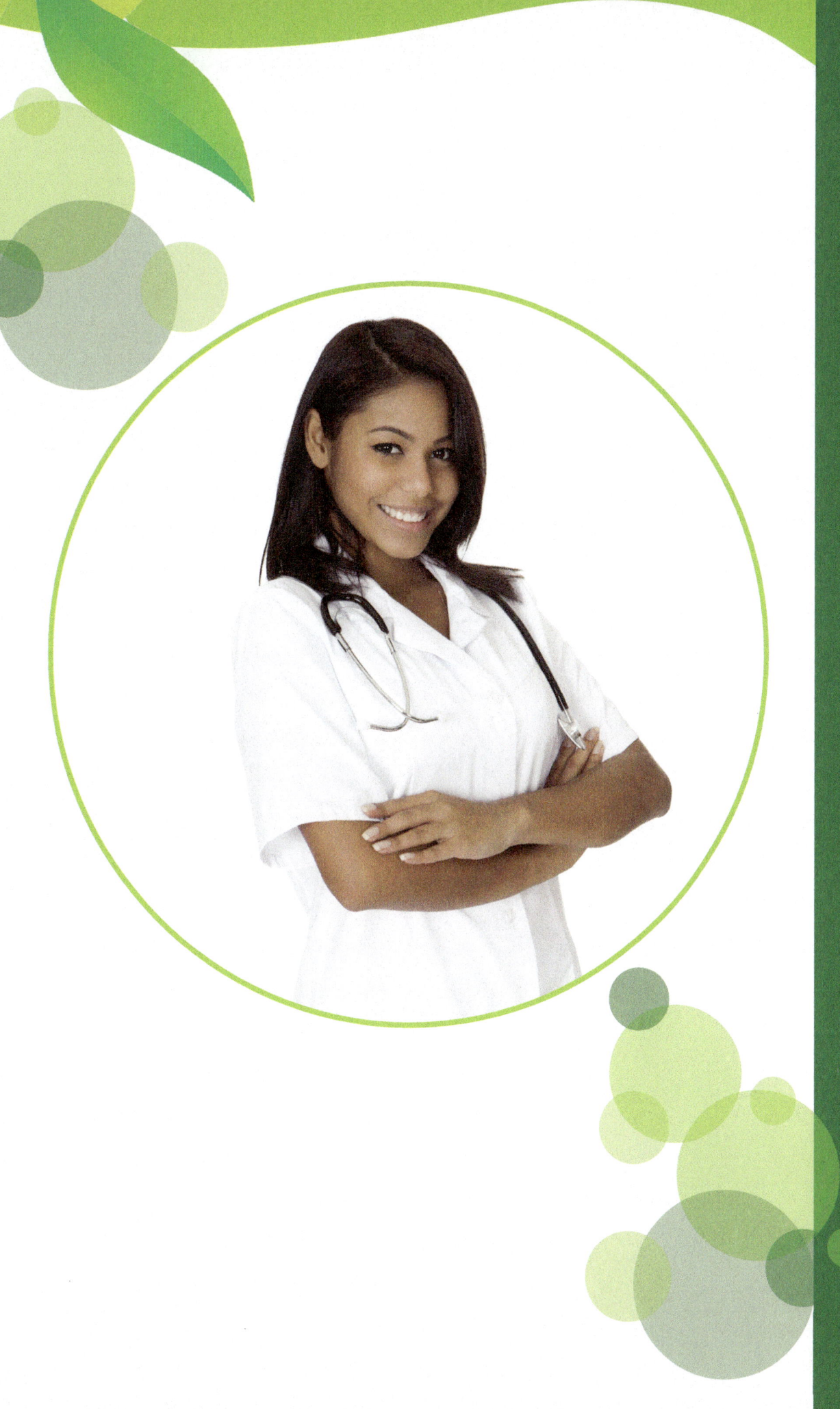

AROMATHERAPY CLIENT INTAKE FORMS

ACP-1 ACTIVITY: AROMATHERAPY CLIENT INTAKE FORM

In this course, we covered making aromatic and therapeutic blends for treating sicknesses and diseases. You will find most people are interested in finding answers to their health concerns and are seeking an alternative to prescribed medicines. As you have learned, therapeutic grade essential oils do offer us a great option to meds!

For those who would like to pursue a career in aromatherapy as a Certified Aromatherapist, performing a case study will give you an opportunity to start your practice. In this activity, you will use this intake form just like you would if you were practicing clinical aromatherapy.

Use this form to collect data for your client (this can be yourself or a friend). It is important to get as much health history as possible in guiding users on which essential oils will benefit them. With this information, write up a case study (using the 2nd form that follows) for a prescribed treatment plan using essential oils. Feel free to ad lib if you do not have a "health issue" or a friend willing to volunteer.

Aromatherapy Intake Form

First Name: _____ Last Name: _____

Date of Birth: _____ / _____ / _____

Address: _____

_____

City: _____ State: _____ Zip: _____

Phone Number: _____ Email: _____

1. *How would you describe your overall health?*

_____
_____
_____
_____
_____

2. *What are you hoping essential oils can do for your health?*

_____
_____
_____
_____

3. *Do you have any chronic illnesses? If yes, what type of condition?*

_____
_____
_____
_____

4. *How long have you been aware of this condition?*

_____
_____
_____
_____

5. *What type of treatment(s) have you tried?*

_____
_____
_____
_____

6. *What has helped?*

_____
_____
_____
_____

7. *What symptoms are most difficult for you?*

_____
_____
_____
_____

8. *Do you have any acute conditions you would like to address?*

_____
_____
_____
_____

9. *Please list any allergies:*

_____   _____
_____   _____
_____   _____

10. *Are you pregnant or trying to become pregnant?*   Yes ☐   No ☐

11. *Do you have epilepsy?*   Yes ☐   No ☐

12. *Do you have high/low blood pressure?*   Yes ☐   No ☐

13. *Which oils or aromas are you drawn to?*

_____   _____
_____   _____
_____   _____

14. *Do any oils or aromas disturb you?*

_____
_____
_____
_____

15. *Are you under the care of a physician? If so, please list the condition(s) you are being treated for:*

_____
_____
_____
_____

16. *Please list any medications you are taking:*

_____   _____
_____   _____
_____   _____
_____   _____

Since essential oils should not be used under certain circumstances, I affirm that I have truthfully answered all questions pertaining to my health on the Aromatherapy Intake Form. *Please sign below.*

Signature:_____

Date: _____ / _____ / _____

Aromatherapy Clinical Practice Intake Notes

For your aromatherapy clinical practice, you will need to make intake notes for each client.
Use this form as a guide to help you get started.

Client Profile & Lifestyle

TIP — *Here you can write a summary of what is covered in the consultation form. You should be able to see from the client's lifestyle what is causing any particular problem, i.e. a lot of driving could lead to backache. You need detailed information about the client to treat them holistically.*

Treatment Plan

TIP — *Here you can explain what the client would like you to help them with. For example, do they have a bad back? You would choose oils that help relieve aches and pains, or are antispasmodic. Will your plan be focusing on any particular area of the body?*

Treatment One

Refer to Lesson 10: Carrier Oils for determining which oils are best for certain conditions.

Details of How The Treatment Was Conducted

TIP — *What methods were recommended in essential oil usage?*

Details of How The Client Felt Before, During and After The Treatment

TIP — *Here you can point out the client's disposition, and/or any physical/emotional problems they have.*

Home Care and After Care Advice

TIP — *Note recommended methods for self-treatments i.e. baths, compresses, etc. with quantities of oil and frequency of use. Advise client of normal reactions to treatments — such as feeling tired, etc. Inform client of any aftereffects of oils i.e. phototoxic so stay out of the sun.*

Reflective Practice

TIP — *How did you perform as a therapist? Were you nervous/confident?*

Treatment Follow Up

TIP — *Check your consultation form for any changes since initial visit. Make sure that the client has not become pregnant, has had any bad reactions, or is on any new medications, etc.*

Overall Conclusion

TIP — *Did your recommendations accomplish their goals? Did you learn anything from treating this client? Would you have done anything differently?*

ACP-1 ACTIVITY: AROMATHERAPY CLIENT INTAKE FORM

In this course, we covered making aromatic and therapeutic blends for treating sicknesses and diseases. You will find most people are interested in finding answers to their health concerns and are seeking an alternative to prescribed medicines. As you have learned, therapeutic grade essential oils do offer us a great option to meds!

For those who would like to pursue a career in aromatherapy as a Certified Aromatherapist, performing a case study will give you an opportunity to start your practice. In this activity, you will use this intake form just like you would if you were practicing clinical aromatherapy.

Use this form to collect data for your client (this can be yourself or a friend). It is important to get as much health history as possible in guiding users on which essential oils will benefit them. With this information, write up a case study (using the 2nd form that follows) for a prescribed treatment plan using essential oils. Feel free to ad lib if you do not have a "health issue" or a friend willing to volunteer.

Aromatherapy Intake Form

First Name: _____ Last Name: _____

Date of Birth: _____ / _____ / _____

Address: _____

_____

City: _____ State: _____ Zip: _____

Phone Number: _____ Email: _____

1. *How would you describe your overall health?*

_____
_____
_____
_____
_____

2. *What are you hoping essential oils can do for your health?*

_____
_____
_____
_____

3. *Do you have any chronic illnesses? If yes, what type of condition?*

_____
_____
_____
_____

4. *How long have you been aware of this condition?*

_____
_____
_____
_____

5. *What type of treatment(s) have you tried?*

_____
_____
_____
_____

6. *What has helped?*

_____
_____
_____
_____

7. *What symptoms are most difficult for you?*

_____
_____
_____
_____

8. *Do you have any acute conditions you would like to address?*

_____
_____
_____
_____

9. *Please list any allergies:*

_____   _____
_____   _____
_____   _____
_____   _____

10. *Are you pregnant or trying to become pregnant?*   Yes [ ]   No [ ]

11. *Do you have epilepsy?*   Yes [ ]   No [ ]

12. *Do you have high/low blood pressure?*   Yes [ ]   No [ ]

13. *Which oils or aromas are you drawn to?*

_____   _____
_____   _____
_____   _____
_____   _____

14. *Do any oils or aromas disturb you?*

_____
_____
_____
_____

15. *Are you under the care of a physician? If so, please list the condition(s) you are being treated for:*

_____
_____
_____
_____

16. *Please list any medications you are taking:*

_____   _____
_____   _____
_____   _____
_____   _____

Since essential oils should not be used under certain circumstances, I affirm that I have truthfully answered all questions pertaining to my health on the Aromatherapy Intake Form. *Please sign below.*

Signature:_____

Date: _____ / _____ / _____

Aromatherapy Clinical Practice Intake Notes

For your aromatherapy clinical practice, you will need to make intake notes for each client. Use this form as a guide to help you get started.

Client Profile & Lifestyle

TIP — *Here you can write a summary of what is covered in the consultation form. You should be able to see from the client's lifestyle what is causing any particular problem, i.e. a lot of driving could lead to backache. You need detailed information about the client to treat them holistically.*

Treatment Plan

TIP — *Here you can explain what the client would like you to help them with. For example, do they have a bad back? You would choose oils that help relieve aches and pains, or are antispasmodic. Will your plan be focusing on any particular area of the body?*

Treatment One

Refer to Lesson 10: Carrier Oils for determining which oils are best for certain conditions.

Details of How The Treatment Was Conducted

TIP — *What methods were recommended in essential oil usage?*

Details of How The Client Felt Before, During and After The Treatment

TIP — *Here you can point out the client's disposition, and/or any physical/emotional problems they have.*

Home Care and After Care Advice

TIP — *Note recommended methods for self-treatments i.e. baths, compresses, etc. with quantities of oil and frequency of use. Advise client of normal reactions to treatments — such as feeling tired, etc. Inform client of any aftereffects of oils i.e. phototoxic so stay out of the sun.*

Reflective Practice

TIP — *How did you perform as a therapist? Were you nervous/confident?*

Treatment Follow Up

TIP — *Check your consultation form for any changes since initial visit. Make sure that the client has not become pregnant, has had any bad reactions, or is on any new medications, etc.*

Overall Conclusion

TIP — *Did your recommendations accomplish their goals? Did you learn anything from treating this client? Would you have done anything differently?*

ACP-1 ACTIVITY: AROMATHERAPY CLIENT INTAKE FORM

In this course, we covered making aromatic and therapeutic blends for treating sicknesses and diseases. You will find most people are interested in finding answers to their health concerns and are seeking an alternative to prescribed medicines. As you have learned, therapeutic grade essential oils do offer us a great option to meds!

For those who would like to pursue a career in aromatherapy as a Certified Aromatherapist, performing a case study will give you an opportunity to start your practice. In this activity, you will use this intake form just like you would if you were practicing clinical aromatherapy.

Use this form to collect data for your client (this can be yourself or a friend). It is important to get as much health history as possible in guiding users on which essential oils will benefit them. With this information, write up a case study (using the 2nd form that follows) for a prescribed treatment plan using essential oils. Feel free to ad lib if you do not have a "health issue" or a friend willing to volunteer.

Aromatherapy Intake Form

First Name: _____ Last Name: _____

Date of Birth: _____ / _____ / _____

Address: _____
_____

City: _____ State: _____ Zip: _____

Phone Number: _____ Email: _____

1. *How would you describe your overall health?*

_____
_____
_____
_____
_____

2. *What are you hoping essential oils can do for your health?*

_____
_____
_____
_____

3. *Do you have any chronic illnesses? If yes, what type of condition?*

_____
_____
_____
_____

4. *How long have you been aware of this condition?*

_____
_____
_____
_____

5. *What type of treatment(s) have you tried?*

_____
_____
_____
_____

6. *What has helped?*

_____
_____
_____
_____

7. *What symptoms are most difficult for you?*

_____
_____
_____
_____

8. *Do you have any acute conditions you would like to address?*

_____
_____
_____
_____

9. *Please list any allergies:*

_____   _____
_____   _____
_____   _____
_____   _____

10. *Are you pregnant or trying to become pregnant?*   Yes ☐   No ☐

11. *Do you have epilepsy?*   Yes ☐   No ☐

12. *Do you have high/low blood pressure?*   Yes ☐   No ☐

13. *Which oils or aromas are you drawn to?*

_____   _____
_____   _____
_____   _____
_____   _____

14. *Do any oils or aromas disturb you?*

_____
_____
_____
_____

15. *Are you under the care of a physician? If so, please list the condition(s) you are being treated for:*

_____
_____
_____
_____

16. *Please list any medications you are taking:*

_____	_____
_____	_____
_____	_____

Since essential oils should not be used under certain circumstances, I affirm that I have truthfully answered all questions pertaining to my health on the Aromatherapy Intake Form. *Please sign below.*

Signature:_____

Date:_____ / _____ / _____

Aromatherapy Clinical Practice Intake Notes

For your aromatherapy clinical practice, you will need to make intake notes for each client. Use this form as a guide to help you get started.

Client Profile & Lifestyle

TIP — *Here you can write a summary of what is covered in the consultation form. You should be able to see from the client's lifestyle what is causing any particular problem, i.e. a lot of driving could lead to backache. You need detailed information about the client to treat them holistically.*

Treatment Plan

TIP — *Here you can explain what the client would like you to help them with. For example, do they have a bad back? You would choose oils that help relieve aches and pains, or are antispasmodic. Will your plan be focusing on any particular area of the body?*

Treatment One

Refer to Lesson 10: Carrier Oils for determining which oils are best for certain conditions.

Details of How The Treatment Was Conducted

TIP — *What methods were recommended in essential oil usage?*

Details of How The Client Felt Before, During and After The Treatment

TIP — *Here you can point out the client's disposition, and/or any physical/emotional problems they have.*

Home Care and After Care Advice

TIP — *Note recommended methods for self-treatments i.e. baths, compresses, etc. with quantities of oil and frequency of use. Advise client of normal reactions to treatments — such as feeling tired, etc. Inform client of any aftereffects of oils i.e. phototoxic so stay out of the sun.*

Reflective Practice

TIP — *How did you perform as a therapist? Were you nervous/confident?*

Treatment Follow Up

TIP — *Check your consultation form for any changes since initial visit. Make sure that the client has not become pregnant, has had any bad reactions, or is on any new medications, etc.*

Overall Conclusion

TIP — *Did your recommendations accomplish their goals? Did you learn anything from treating this client? Would you have done anything differently?*

ACP-1 ACTIVITY: AROMATHERAPY CLIENT INTAKE FORM

In this course, we covered making aromatic and therapeutic blends for treating sicknesses and diseases. You will find most people are interested in finding answers to their health concerns and are seeking an alternative to prescribed medicines. As you have learned, therapeutic grade essential oils do offer us a great option to meds!

For those who would like to pursue a career in aromatherapy as a Certified Aromatherapist, performing a case study will give you an opportunity to start your practice. In this activity, you will use this intake form just like you would if you were practicing clinical aromatherapy.

Use this form to collect data for your client (this can be yourself or a friend). It is important to get as much health history as possible in guiding users on which essential oils will benefit them. With this information, write up a case study (using the 2nd form that follows) for a prescribed treatment plan using essential oils. Feel free to ad lib if you do not have a "health issue" or a friend willing to volunteer.

Aromatherapy Intake Form

First Name: _____ Last Name: _____

Date of Birth: _____ / _____ / _____

Address: _____

_____

City: _____ State: _____ Zip: _____

Phone Number: _____ Email: _____

1. *How would you describe your overall health?*

_____

_____

_____

_____

2. What are you hoping essential oils can do for your health?
___
___
___
___

3. Do you have any chronic illnesses? If yes, what type of condition?
___
___
___
___

4. How long have you been aware of this condition?
___
___
___
___

5. What type of treatment(s) have you tried?
___
___
___
___

6. What has helped?
___
___
___
___

7. *What symptoms are most difficult for you?*

_____
_____
_____
_____

8. *Do you have any acute conditions you would like to address?*

_____
_____
_____
_____

9. *Please list any allergies:*

_____ _____
_____ _____
_____ _____
_____ _____

10. *Are you pregnant or trying to become pregnant?*   Yes ☐   No ☐

11. *Do you have epilepsy?*   Yes ☐   No ☐

12. *Do you have high/low blood pressure?*   Yes ☐   No ☐

13. *Which oils or aromas are you drawn to?*

_____ _____
_____ _____
_____ _____
_____ _____

14. *Do any oils or aromas disturb you?*

_____
_____
_____
_____

15. *Are you under the care of a physician? If so, please list the condition(s) you are being treated for:*

_____
_____
_____
_____

16. *Please list any medications you are taking:*

_____   _____
_____   _____
_____   _____
_____   _____

Since essential oils should not be used under certain circumstances, I affirm that I have truthfully answered all questions pertaining to my health on the Aromatherapy Intake Form. *Please sign below.*

Signature:_____

Date: _____ / _____ / _____

Aromatherapy Clinical Practice Intake Notes

For your aromatherapy clinical practice, you will need to make intake notes for each client. Use this form as a guide to help you get started.

Client Profile & Lifestyle

TIP — *Here you can write a summary of what is covered in the consultation form. You should be able to see from the client's lifestyle what is causing any particular problem, i.e. a lot of driving could lead to backache. You need detailed information about the client to treat them holistically.*

Treatment Plan

TIP — *Here you can explain what the client would like you to help them with. For example, do they have a bad back? You would choose oils that help relieve aches and pains, or are antispasmodic. Will your plan be focusing on any particular area of the body?*

Treatment One

Refer to Lesson 10: Carrier Oils for determining which oils are best for certain conditions.

Details of How The Treatment Was Conducted

TIP — *What methods were recommended in essential oil usage?*

Details of How The Client Felt Before, During and After The Treatment

TIP — *Here you can point out the client's disposition, and/or any physical/emotional problems they have.*

Home Care and After Care Advice

TIP — *Note recommended methods for self-treatments i.e. baths, compresses, etc. with quantities of oil and frequency of use. Advise client of normal reactions to treatments — such as feeling tired, etc. Inform client of any aftereffects of oils i.e. phototoxic so stay out of the sun.*

Reflective Practice

TIP — *How did you perform as a therapist? Were you nervous/confident?*

Treatment Follow Up

TIP — *Check your consultation form for any changes since initial visit. Make sure that the client has not become pregnant, has had any bad reactions, or is on any new medications, etc.*

Overall Conclusion

TIP — *Did your recommendations accomplish their goals? Did you learn anything from treating this client? Would you have done anything differently?*

ACP-1 ACTIVITY: AROMATHERAPY CLIENT INTAKE FORM

In this course, we covered making aromatic and therapeutic blends for treating sicknesses and diseases. You will find most people are interested in finding answers to their health concerns and are seeking an alternative to prescribed medicines. As you have learned, therapeutic grade essential oils do offer us a great option to meds!

For those who would like to pursue a career in aromatherapy as a Certified Aromatherapist, performing a case study will give you an opportunity to start your practice. In this activity, you will use this intake form just like you would if you were practicing clinical aromatherapy.

Use this form to collect data for your client (this can be yourself or a friend). It is important to get as much health history as possible in guiding users on which essential oils will benefit them. With this information, write up a case study (using the 2nd form that follows) for a prescribed treatment plan using essential oils. Feel free to ad lib if you do not have a "health issue" or a friend willing to volunteer.

Aromatherapy Intake Form

First Name: _____ Last Name: _____

Date of Birth: _____ / _____ / _____

Address: _____

_____

City: _____ State: _____ Zip: _____

Phone Number: _____ Email: _____

1. *How would you describe your overall health?*

_____
_____
_____
_____
_____

2. *What are you hoping essential oils can do for your health?*

_____
_____
_____
_____

3. *Do you have any chronic illnesses? If yes, what type of condition?*

_____
_____
_____
_____

4. *How long have you been aware of this condition?*

_____
_____
_____
_____

5. *What type of treatment(s) have you tried?*

_____
_____
_____
_____

6. *What has helped?*

_____
_____
_____
_____

7. *What symptoms are most difficult for you?*

_____
_____
_____
_____

8. *Do you have any acute conditions you would like to address?*

_____
_____
_____
_____

9. *Please list any allergies:*

_____   _____
_____   _____
_____   _____
_____   _____

10. *Are you pregnant or trying to become pregnant?*   Yes ☐   No ☐

11. *Do you have epilepsy?*   Yes ☐   No ☐

12. *Do you have high/low blood pressure?*   Yes ☐   No ☐

13. *Which oils or aromas are you drawn to?*

_____   _____
_____   _____
_____   _____
_____   _____

14. *Do any oils or aromas disturb you?*

_____
_____
_____
_____

15. *Are you under the care of a physician? If so, please list the condition(s) you are being treated for:*

_____
_____
_____
_____

16. *Please list any medications you are taking:*

_____   _____
_____   _____
_____   _____
_____   _____

Since essential oils should not be used under certain circumstances, I affirm that I have truthfully answered all questions pertaining to my health on the Aromatherapy Intake Form. *Please sign below.*

Signature:_____

Date: _____ / _____ / _____

Aromatherapy Clinical Practice Intake Notes

For your aromatherapy clinical practice, you will need to make intake notes for each client.
Use this form as a guide to help you get started.

Client Profile & Lifestyle

TIP — *Here you can write a summary of what is covered in the consultation form. You should be able to see from the client's lifestyle what is causing any particular problem, i.e. a lot of driving could lead to backache. You need detailed information about the client to treat them holistically.*

Treatment Plan

TIP — *Here you can explain what the client would like you to help them with. For example, do they have a bad back? You would choose oils that help relieve aches and pains, or are antispasmodic. Will your plan be focusing on any particular area of the body?*

Treatment One

Refer to Lesson 10: Carrier Oils for determining which oils are best for certain conditions.

Details of How The Treatment Was Conducted

TIP — *What methods were recommended in essential oil usage?*

Details of How The Client Felt Before, During and After The Treatment

TIP — *Here you can point out the client's disposition, and/or any physical/emotional problems they have.*

Home Care and After Care Advice

TIP — *Note recommended methods for self-treatments i.e. baths, compresses, etc. with quantities of oil and frequency of use. Advise client of normal reactions to treatments — such as feeling tired, etc. Inform client of any aftereffects of oils i.e. phototoxic so stay out of the sun.*

Reflective Practice

TIP — *How did you perform as a therapist? Were you nervous/confident?*

Treatment Follow Up

TIP — *Check your consultation form for any changes since initial visit. Make sure that the client has not become pregnant, has had any bad reactions, or is on any new medications, etc.*

Overall Conclusion

TIP — *Did your recommendations accomplish their goals? Did you learn anything from treating this client? Would you have done anything differently?*

ACP-1 ACTIVITY: AROMATHERAPY CLIENT INTAKE FORM

In this course, we covered making aromatic and therapeutic blends for treating sicknesses and diseases. You will find most people are interested in finding answers to their health concerns and are seeking an alternative to prescribed medicines. As you have learned, therapeutic grade essential oils do offer us a great option to meds!

For those who would like to pursue a career in aromatherapy as a Certified Aromatherapist, performing a case study will give you an opportunity to start your practice. In this activity, you will use this intake form just like you would if you were practicing clinical aromatherapy.

Use this form to collect data for your client (this can be yourself or a friend). It is important to get as much health history as possible in guiding users on which essential oils will benefit them. With this information, write up a case study (using the 2nd form that follows) for a prescribed treatment plan using essential oils. Feel free to ad lib if you do not have a "health issue" or a friend willing to volunteer.

Aromatherapy Intake Form

First Name: _____ Last Name: _____

Date of Birth: _____ / _____ / _____

Address: _____
_____

City: _____ State: _____ Zip: _____

Phone Number: _____ Email: _____

1. *How would you describe your overall health?*

_____
_____
_____
_____
_____

2. *What are you hoping essential oils can do for your health?*
___

3. *Do you have any chronic illnesses? If yes, what type of condition?*
___

4. *How long have you been aware of this condition?*
___

5. *What type of treatment(s) have you tried?*
___

6. *What has helped?*
___

7. *What symptoms are most difficult for you?*

_____
_____
_____
_____

8. *Do you have any acute conditions you would like to address?*

_____
_____
_____
_____

9. *Please list any allergies:*

_____ _____
_____ _____
_____ _____

10. *Are you pregnant or trying to become pregnant?*   Yes [ ]   No [ ]

11. *Do you have epilepsy?*   Yes [ ]   No [ ]

12. *Do you have high/low blood pressure?*   Yes [ ]   No [ ]

13. *Which oils or aromas are you drawn to?*

_____ _____
_____ _____
_____ _____

14. *Do any oils or aromas disturb you?*

_____
_____
_____
_____

15. *Are you under the care of a physician? If so, please list the condition(s) you are being treated for:*

_____
_____
_____
_____

16. *Please list any medications you are taking:*

_____ _____
_____ _____
_____ _____
_____ _____

Since essential oils should not be used under certain circumstances, I affirm that I have truthfully answered all questions pertaining to my health on the Aromatherapy Intake Form. *Please sign below.*

Signature:_____

Date: _____ / _____ / _____

Aromatherapy Clinical Practice Intake Notes

For your aromatherapy clinical practice, you will need to make intake notes for each client.
Use this form as a guide to help you get started.

Client Profile & Lifestyle

TIP — *Here you can write a summary of what is covered in the consultation form. You should be able to see from the client's lifestyle what is causing any particular problem, i.e. a lot of driving could lead to backache. You need detailed information about the client to treat them holistically.*

Treatment Plan

TIP — *Here you can explain what the client would like you to help them with. For example, do they have a bad back? You would choose oils that help relieve aches and pains, or are antispasmodic. Will your plan be focusing on any particular area of the body?*

Treatment One

*Refer to **Lesson 10: Carrier Oils** for determining which oils are best for certain conditions.*

Details of How The Treatment Was Conducted

TIP — *What methods were recommended in essential oil usage?*

Details of How The Client Felt Before, During and After The Treatment

TIP — *Here you can point out the client's disposition, and/or any physical/emotional problems they have.*

Home Care and After Care Advice

TIP — *Note recommended methods for self-treatments i.e. baths, compresses, etc. with quantities of oil and frequency of use. Advise client of normal reactions to treatments — such as feeling tired, etc. Inform client of any aftereffects of oils i.e. phototoxic so stay out of the sun.*

Reflective Practice

TIP — *How did you perform as a therapist? Were you nervous/confident?*

Treatment Follow Up

TIP — *Check your consultation form for any changes since initial visit. Make sure that the client has not become pregnant, has had any bad reactions, or is on any new medications, etc.*

Overall Conclusion

TIP — *Did your recommendations accomplish their goals? Did you learn anything from treating this client? Would you have done anything differently?*

ACP-1 ACTIVITY: AROMATHERAPY CLIENT INTAKE FORM

In this course, we covered making aromatic and therapeutic blends for treating sicknesses and diseases. You will find most people are interested in finding answers to their health concerns and are seeking an alternative to prescribed medicines. As you have learned, therapeutic grade essential oils do offer us a great option to meds!

For those who would like to pursue a career in aromatherapy as a Certified Aromatherapist, performing a case study will give you an opportunity to start your practice. In this activity, you will use this intake form just like you would if you were practicing clinical aromatherapy.

Use this form to collect data for your client (this can be yourself or a friend). It is important to get as much health history as possible in guiding users on which essential oils will benefit them. With this information, write up a case study (using the 2nd form that follows) for a prescribed treatment plan using essential oils. Feel free to ad lib if you do not have a "health issue" or a friend willing to volunteer.

Aromatherapy Intake Form

First Name: _____ Last Name: _____

Date of Birth: _____ / _____ / _____

Address: _____

_____

City: _____ State: _____ Zip: _____

Phone Number: _____ Email: _____

1. *How would you describe your overall health?*

_____
_____
_____
_____
_____

2. What are you hoping essential oils can do for your health?
_____
_____
_____
_____

3. Do you have any chronic illnesses? If yes, what type of condition?
_____
_____
_____
_____

4. How long have you been aware of this condition?
_____
_____
_____
_____

5. What type of treatment(s) have you tried?
_____
_____
_____
_____

6. What has helped?
_____
_____
_____
_____

7. *What symptoms are most difficult for you?*

_____
_____
_____
_____

8. *Do you have any acute conditions you would like to address?*

_____
_____
_____
_____

9. *Please list any allergies:*

_____   _____
_____   _____
_____   _____
_____   _____

10. *Are you pregnant or trying to become pregnant?*   Yes ☐   No ☐

11. *Do you have epilepsy?*   Yes ☐   No ☐

12. *Do you have high/low blood pressure?*   Yes ☐   No ☐

13. *Which oils or aromas are you drawn to?*

_____   _____
_____   _____
_____   _____
_____   _____

14. *Do any oils or aromas disturb you?*

_____
_____
_____
_____

15. *Are you under the care of a physician? If so, please list the condition(s) you are being treated for:*

_____
_____
_____
_____

16. *Please list any medications you are taking:*

_____   _____
_____   _____
_____   _____
_____   _____

Since essential oils should not be used under certain circumstances, I affirm that I have truthfully answered all questions pertaining to my health on the Aromatherapy Intake Form. *Please sign below.*

Signature:_____

Date: _____ / _____ / _____

Aromatherapy Clinical Practice Intake Notes

For your aromatherapy clinical practice, you will need to make intake notes for each client.
Use this form as a guide to help you get started.

Client Profile & Lifestyle

TIP — *Here you can write a summary of what is covered in the consultation form. You should be able to see from the client's lifestyle what is causing any particular problem, i.e. a lot of driving could lead to backache. You need detailed information about the client to treat them holistically.*

Treatment Plan

TIP — *Here you can explain what the client would like you to help them with. For example, do they have a bad back? You would choose oils that help relieve aches and pains, or are antispasmodic. Will your plan be focusing on any particular area of the body?*

Treatment One

Refer to Lesson 10: Carrier Oils for determining which oils are best for certain conditions.

Details of How The Treatment Was Conducted

TIP — *What methods were recommended in essential oil usage?*

Details of How The Client Felt Before, During and After The Treatment

TIP — *Here you can point out the client's disposition, and/or any physical/emotional problems they have.*

Home Care and After Care Advice

TIP — *Note recommended methods for self-treatments i.e. baths, compresses, etc. with quantities of oil and frequency of use. Advise client of normal reactions to treatments — such as feeling tired, etc. Inform client of any aftereffects of oils i.e. phototoxic so stay out of the sun.*

Reflective Practice

TIP — *How did you perform as a therapist? Were you nervous/confident?*

Treatment Follow Up

TIP — *Check your consultation form for any changes since initial visit. Make sure that the client has not become pregnant, has had any bad reactions, or is on any new medications, etc.*

Overall Conclusion

TIP — *Did your recommendations accomplish their goals? Did you learn anything from treating this client? Would you have done anything differently?*

ACP-1 ACTIVITY: AROMATHERAPY CLIENT INTAKE FORM

In this course, we covered making aromatic and therapeutic blends for treating sicknesses and diseases. You will find most people are interested in finding answers to their health concerns and are seeking an alternative to prescribed medicines. As you have learned, therapeutic grade essential oils do offer us a great option to meds!

For those who would like to pursue a career in aromatherapy as a Certified Aromatherapist, performing a case study will give you an opportunity to start your practice. In this activity, you will use this intake form just like you would if you were practicing clinical aromatherapy.

Use this form to collect data for your client (this can be yourself or a friend). It is important to get as much health history as possible in guiding users on which essential oils will benefit them. With this information, write up a case study (using the 2nd form that follows) for a prescribed treatment plan using essential oils. Feel free to ad lib if you do not have a "health issue" or a friend willing to volunteer.

Aromatherapy Intake Form

First Name: _____ Last Name: _____

Date of Birth: _____ / _____ / _____

Address: _____

_____

City: _____ State: _____ Zip: _____

Phone Number: _____ Email: _____

1. *How would you describe your overall health?*

_____
_____
_____
_____
_____

2. What are you hoping essential oils can do for your health?
_____
_____
_____
_____

3. Do you have any chronic illnesses? If yes, what type of condition?
_____
_____
_____
_____

4. How long have you been aware of this condition?
_____
_____
_____
_____

5. What type of treatment(s) have you tried?
_____
_____
_____
_____

6. What has helped?
_____
_____
_____
_____

7. *What symptoms are most difficult for you?*

_____
_____
_____
_____

8. *Do you have any acute conditions you would like to address?*

_____
_____
_____
_____

9. *Please list any allergies:*

_____   _____
_____   _____
_____   _____

10. *Are you pregnant or trying to become pregnant?*   Yes ☐   No ☐

11. *Do you have epilepsy?*   Yes ☐   No ☐

12. *Do you have high/low blood pressure?*   Yes ☐   No ☐

13. *Which oils or aromas are you drawn to?*

_____   _____
_____   _____
_____   _____

14. *Do any oils or aromas disturb you?*

_____
_____
_____
_____

15. *Are you under the care of a physician? If so, please list the condition(s) you are being treated for:*

_____
_____
_____
_____

16. *Please list any medications you are taking:*

_____   _____
_____   _____
_____   _____
_____   _____

Since essential oils should not be used under certain circumstances, I affirm that I have truthfully answered all questions pertaining to my health on the Aromatherapy Intake Form. *Please sign below.*

Signature:_____

Date: _____ / _____ / _____

Aromatherapy Clinical Practice Intake Notes

For your aromatherapy clinical practice, you will need to make intake notes for each client. Use this form as a guide to help you get started.

Client Profile & Lifestyle

> **TIP** — *Here you can write a summary of what is covered in the consultation form. You should be able to see from the client's lifestyle what is causing any particular problem, i.e. a lot of driving could lead to backache. You need detailed information about the client to treat them holistically.*

Treatment Plan

> **TIP** — *Here you can explain what the client would like you to help them with. For example, do they have a bad back? You would choose oils that help relieve aches and pains, or are antispasmodic. Will your plan be focusing on any particular area of the body?*

Treatment One

Refer to Lesson 10: Carrier Oils for determining which oils are best for certain conditions.

Details of How The Treatment Was Conducted

TIP — *What methods were recommended in essential oil usage?*

Details of How The Client Felt Before, During and After The Treatment

TIP — *Here you can point out the client's disposition, and/or any physical/emotional problems they have.*

Home Care and After Care Advice

TIP — *Note recommended methods for self-treatments i.e. baths, compresses, etc. with quantities of oil and frequency of use. Advise client of normal reactions to treatments — such as feeling tired, etc. Inform client of any aftereffects of oils i.e. phototoxic so stay out of the sun.*

Reflective Practice

TIP — *How did you perform as a therapist? Were you nervous/confident?*

Treatment Follow Up

TIP — *Check your consultation form for any changes since initial visit. Make sure that the client has not become pregnant, has had any bad reactions, or is on any new medications, etc.*

Overall Conclusion

TIP — *Did your recommendations accomplish their goals? Did you learn anything from treating this client? Would you have done anything differently?*

ACP-1 ACTIVITY: AROMATHERAPY CLIENT INTAKE FORM

In this course, we covered making aromatic and therapeutic blends for treating sicknesses and diseases. You will find most people are interested in finding answers to their health concerns and are seeking an alternative to prescribed medicines. As you have learned, therapeutic grade essential oils do offer us a great option to meds!

For those who would like to pursue a career in aromatherapy as a Certified Aromatherapist, performing a case study will give you an opportunity to start your practice. In this activity, you will use this intake form just like you would if you were practicing clinical aromatherapy.

Use this form to collect data for your client (this can be yourself or a friend). It is important to get as much health history as possible in guiding users on which essential oils will benefit them. With this information, write up a case study (using the 2nd form that follows) for a prescribed treatment plan using essential oils. Feel free to ad lib if you do not have a "health issue" or a friend willing to volunteer.

Aromatherapy Intake Form

First Name: _____ Last Name: _____

Date of Birth: _____ / _____ / _____

Address: _____
_____

City: _____ State: _____ Zip: _____

Phone Number: _____ Email: _____

1. *How would you describe your overall health?*

_____
_____
_____
_____
_____

2. *What are you hoping essential oils can do for your health?*

_____
_____
_____
_____

3. *Do you have any chronic illnesses? If yes, what type of condition?*

_____
_____
_____
_____

4. *How long have you been aware of this condition?*

_____
_____
_____
_____

5. *What type of treatment(s) have you tried?*

_____
_____
_____
_____

6. *What has helped?*

_____
_____
_____
_____

7. *What symptoms are most difficult for you?*

_____
_____
_____
_____

8. *Do you have any acute conditions you would like to address?*

_____
_____
_____
_____

9. *Please list any allergies:*

_____   _____
_____   _____
_____   _____

10. *Are you pregnant or trying to become pregnant?*   Yes ☐   No ☐

11. *Do you have epilepsy?*   Yes ☐   No ☐

12. *Do you have high/low blood pressure?*   Yes ☐   No ☐

13. *Which oils or aromas are you drawn to?*

_____   _____
_____   _____
_____   _____
_____   _____

14. *Do any oils or aromas disturb you?*

_____
_____
_____
_____

15. *Are you under the care of a physician? If so, please list the condition(s) you are being treated for:*

_____
_____
_____
_____

16. *Please list any medications you are taking:*

_____   _____
_____   _____
_____   _____
_____   _____

Since essential oils should not be used under certain circumstances, I affirm that I have truthfully answered all questions pertaining to my health on the Aromatherapy Intake Form. *Please sign below.*

Signature:_____

Date:_____ / _____ / _____

Aromatherapy Clinical Practice Intake Notes

For your aromatherapy clinical practice, you will need to make intake notes for each client.
Use this form as a guide to help you get started.

Client Profile & Lifestyle

TIP — *Here you can write a summary of what is covered in the consultation form. You should be able to see from the client's lifestyle what is causing any particular problem, i.e. a lot of driving could lead to backache. You need detailed information about the client to treat them holistically.*

Treatment Plan

TIP — *Here you can explain what the client would like you to help them with. For example, do they have a bad back? You would choose oils that help relieve aches and pains, or are antispasmodic. Will your plan be focusing on any particular area of the body?*

Treatment One

Refer to Lesson 10: Carrier Oils for determining which oils are best for certain conditions.

Details of How The Treatment Was Conducted

TIP — *What methods were recommended in essential oil usage?*

Details of How The Client Felt Before, During and After The Treatment

TIP — *Here you can point out the client's disposition, and/or any physical/emotional problems they have.*

Home Care and After Care Advice

TIP — *Note recommended methods for self-treatments i.e. baths, compresses, etc. with quantities of oil and frequency of use. Advise client of normal reactions to treatments — such as feeling tired, etc. Inform client of any aftereffects of oils i.e. phototoxic so stay out of the sun.*

Reflective Practice

TIP — *How did you perform as a therapist? Were you nervous/confident?*

Treatment Follow Up

TIP — *Check your consultation form for any changes since initial visit. Make sure that the client has not become pregnant, has had any bad reactions, or is on any new medications, etc.*

Overall Conclusion

TIP — *Did your recommendations accomplish their goals? Did you learn anything from treating this client? Would you have done anything differently?*

ACP-1 ACTIVITY: AROMATHERAPY CLIENT INTAKE FORM

In this course, we covered making aromatic and therapeutic blends for treating sicknesses and diseases. You will find most people are interested in finding answers to their health concerns and are seeking an alternative to prescribed medicines. As you have learned, therapeutic grade essential oils do offer us a great option to meds!

For those who would like to pursue a career in aromatherapy as a Certified Aromatherapist, performing a case study will give you an opportunity to start your practice. In this activity, you will use this intake form just like you would if you were practicing clinical aromatherapy.

Use this form to collect data for your client (this can be yourself or a friend). It is important to get as much health history as possible in guiding users on which essential oils will benefit them. With this information, write up a case study (using the 2nd form that follows) for a prescribed treatment plan using essential oils. Feel free to ad lib if you do not have a "health issue" or a friend willing to volunteer.

Aromatherapy Intake Form

First Name: _____   Last Name: _____

Date of Birth: _____ / _____ / _____

Address: _____
_____

City: _____   State: _____   Zip: _____

Phone Number: _____   Email: _____

1. *How would you describe your overall health?*

_____
_____
_____
_____
_____

2. *What are you hoping essential oils can do for your health?*
_____
_____
_____
_____

3. *Do you have any chronic illnesses? If yes, what type of condition?*
_____
_____
_____
_____

4. *How long have you been aware of this condition?*
_____
_____
_____
_____

5. *What type of treatment(s) have you tried?*
_____
_____
_____
_____

6. *What has helped?*
_____
_____
_____
_____

7. *What symptoms are most difficult for you?*

_____
_____
_____
_____

8. *Do you have any acute conditions you would like to address?*

_____
_____
_____
_____

9. *Please list any allergies:*

_____ _____
_____ _____
_____ _____

10. *Are you pregnant or trying to become pregnant?*   Yes [   ]   No [   ]

11. *Do you have epilepsy?*   Yes [   ]   No [   ]

12. *Do you have high/low blood pressure?*   Yes [   ]   No [   ]

13. *Which oils or aromas are you drawn to?*

_____ _____
_____ _____
_____ _____

14. *Do any oils or aromas disturb you?*

_____
_____
_____
_____

15. *Are you under the care of a physician? If so, please list the condition(s) you are being treated for:*

_____
_____
_____
_____

16. *Please list any medications you are taking:*

_____ _____
_____ _____
_____ _____
_____ _____

Since essential oils should not be used under certain circumstances, I affirm that I have truthfully answered all questions pertaining to my health on the Aromatherapy Intake Form. *Please sign below.*

Signature: _____

Date: _____ / _____ / _____

Aromatherapy Clinical Practice Intake Notes

For your aromatherapy clinical practice, you will need to make intake notes for each client.
Use this form as a guide to help you get started.

Client Profile & Lifestyle

> **TIP** — *Here you can write a summary of what is covered in the consultation form. You should be able to see from the client's lifestyle what is causing any particular problem, i.e. a lot of driving could lead to backache. You need detailed information about the client to treat them holistically.*

Treatment Plan

> **TIP** — *Here you can explain what the client would like you to help them with. For example, do they have a bad back? You would choose oils that help relieve aches and pains, or are antispasmodic. Will your plan be focusing on any particular area of the body?*

Treatment One

Refer to Lesson 10: Carrier Oils for determining which oils are best for certain conditions.

Details of How The Treatment Was Conducted

TIP — *What methods were recommended in essential oil usage?*

Details of How The Client Felt Before, During and After The Treatment

TIP — *Here you can point out the client's disposition, and/or any physical/emotional problems they have.*

Home Care and After Care Advice

> **TIP** — *Note recommended methods for self-treatments i.e. baths, compresses, etc. with quantities of oil and frequency of use. Advise client of normal reactions to treatments — such as feeling tired, etc. Inform client of any aftereffects of oils i.e. phototoxic so stay out of the sun.*

Reflective Practice

> **TIP** — *How did you perform as a therapist? Were you nervous/confident?*

Treatment Follow Up

TIP — *Check your consultation form for any changes since initial visit. Make sure that the client has not become pregnant, has had any bad reactions, or is on any new medications, etc.*

Overall Conclusion

TIP — *Did your recommendations accomplish their goals? Did you learn anything from treating this client? Would you have done anything differently?*

ACP-1 ACTIVITY: AROMATHERAPY CLIENT INTAKE FORM

In this course, we covered making aromatic and therapeutic blends for treating sicknesses and diseases. You will find most people are interested in finding answers to their health concerns and are seeking an alternative to prescribed medicines. As you have learned, therapeutic grade essential oils do offer us a great option to meds!

For those who would like to pursue a career in aromatherapy as a Certified Aromatherapist, performing a case study will give you an opportunity to start your practice. In this activity, you will use this intake form just like you would if you were practicing clinical aromatherapy.

Use this form to collect data for your client (this can be yourself or a friend). It is important to get as much health history as possible in guiding users on which essential oils will benefit them. With this information, write up a case study (using the 2nd form that follows) for a prescribed treatment plan using essential oils. Feel free to ad lib if you do not have a "health issue" or a friend willing to volunteer.

Aromatherapy Intake Form

First Name: _____ Last Name: _____

Date of Birth: _____ / _____ / _____

Address: _____
_____

City: _____ State: _____ Zip: _____

Phone Number: _____ Email: _____

1. *How would you describe your overall health?*

_____
_____
_____
_____
_____

2. *What are you hoping essential oils can do for your health?*

_____
_____
_____
_____

3. *Do you have any chronic illnesses? If yes, what type of condition?*

_____
_____
_____
_____

4. *How long have you been aware of this condition?*

_____
_____
_____
_____

5. *What type of treatment(s) have you tried?*

_____
_____
_____
_____

6. *What has helped?*

_____
_____
_____
_____

7. *What symptoms are most difficult for you?*

_____
_____
_____
_____

8. *Do you have any acute conditions you would like to address?*

_____
_____
_____
_____

9. *Please list any allergies:*

_____   _____
_____   _____
_____   _____

10. *Are you pregnant or trying to become pregnant?*   Yes ☐   No ☐

11. *Do you have epilepsy?*   Yes ☐   No ☐

12. *Do you have high/low blood pressure?*   Yes ☐   No ☐

13. *Which oils or aromas are you drawn to?*

_____   _____
_____   _____
_____   _____

14. *Do any oils or aromas disturb you?*

_____
_____
_____
_____

15. *Are you under the care of a physician? If so, please list the condition(s) you are being treated for:*

_____
_____
_____
_____

16. *Please list any medications you are taking:*

_____   _____
_____   _____
_____   _____
_____   _____

Since essential oils should not be used under certain circumstances, I affirm that I have truthfully answered all questions pertaining to my health on the Aromatherapy Intake Form. *Please sign below.*

Signature:_____

Date: _____ / _____ / _____

Aromatherapy Clinical Practice Intake Notes

For your aromatherapy clinical practice, you will need to make intake notes for each client.
Use this form as a guide to help you get started.

Client Profile & Lifestyle

TIP — *Here you can write a summary of what is covered in the consultation form. You should be able to see from the client's lifestyle what is causing any particular problem, i.e. a lot of driving could lead to backache. You need detailed information about the client to treat them holistically.*

Treatment Plan

TIP — *Here you can explain what the client would like you to help them with. For example, do they have a bad back? You would choose oils that help relieve aches and pains, or are antispasmodic. Will your plan be focusing on any particular area of the body?*

Treatment One

Refer to Lesson 10: Carrier Oils for determining which oils are best for certain conditions.

Details of How The Treatment Was Conducted

> **TIP** — *What methods were recommended in essential oil usage?*

Details of How The Client Felt Before, During and After The Treatment

> **TIP** — *Here you can point out the client's disposition, and/or any physical/emotional problems they have.*

Home Care and After Care Advice

TIP — *Note recommended methods for self-treatments i.e. baths, compresses, etc. with quantities of oil and frequency of use. Advise client of normal reactions to treatments — such as feeling tired, etc. Inform client of any aftereffects of oils i.e. phototoxic so stay out of the sun.*

Reflective Practice

TIP — *How did you perform as a therapist? Were you nervous/confident?*

Treatment Follow Up

TIP — *Check your consultation form for any changes since initial visit. Make sure that the client has not become pregnant, has had any bad reactions, or is on any new medications, etc.*

Overall Conclusion

TIP — *Did your recommendations accomplish their goals? Did you learn anything from treating this client? Would you have done anything differently?*

ACP-1 ACTIVITY: AROMATHERAPY CLIENT INTAKE FORM

In this course, we covered making aromatic and therapeutic blends for treating sicknesses and diseases. You will find most people are interested in finding answers to their health concerns and are seeking an alternative to prescribed medicines. As you have learned, therapeutic grade essential oils do offer us a great option to meds!

For those who would like to pursue a career in aromatherapy as a Certified Aromatherapist, performing a case study will give you an opportunity to start your practice. In this activity, you will use this intake form just like you would if you were practicing clinical aromatherapy.

Use this form to collect data for your client (this can be yourself or a friend). It is important to get as much health history as possible in guiding users on which essential oils will benefit them. With this information, write up a case study (using the 2nd form that follows) for a prescribed treatment plan using essential oils. Feel free to ad lib if you do not have a "health issue" or a friend willing to volunteer.

Aromatherapy Intake Form

First Name: _____ Last Name: _____

Date of Birth: _____ / _____ / _____

Address: _____
_____

City: _____ State: _____ Zip: _____

Phone Number: _____ Email: _____

1. *How would you describe your overall health?*

_____
_____
_____
_____
_____

2. What are you hoping essential oils can do for your health?
_____
_____
_____
_____

3. Do you have any chronic illnesses? If yes, what type of condition?
_____
_____
_____
_____

4. How long have you been aware of this condition?
_____
_____
_____
_____

5. What type of treatment(s) have you tried?
_____
_____
_____
_____

6. What has helped?
_____
_____
_____
_____

7. *What symptoms are most difficult for you?*
_____
_____
_____
_____

8. *Do you have any acute conditions you would like to address?*
_____
_____
_____
_____

9. *Please list any allergies:*

_____   _____
_____   _____
_____   _____
_____   _____

10. *Are you pregnant or trying to become pregnant?*   Yes ☐   No ☐

11. *Do you have epilepsy?*   Yes ☐   No ☐

12. *Do you have high/low blood pressure?*   Yes ☐   No ☐

13. *Which oils or aromas are you drawn to?*

_____   _____
_____   _____
_____   _____
_____   _____

14. *Do any oils or aromas disturb you?*

_____
_____
_____
_____

15. *Are you under the care of a physician? If so, please list the condition(s) you are being treated for:*

_____
_____
_____
_____

16. *Please list any medications you are taking:*

_____ _____
_____ _____
_____ _____

Since essential oils should not be used under certain circumstances, I affirm that I have truthfully answered all questions pertaining to my health on the Aromatherapy Intake Form. *Please sign below.*

Signature:_____

Date: _____ / _____ / _____

Aromatherapy Clinical Practice Intake Notes

For your aromatherapy clinical practice, you will need to make intake notes for each client.
Use this form as a guide to help you get started.

Client Profile & Lifestyle

> **TIP** — *Here you can write a summary of what is covered in the consultation form. You should be able to see from the client's lifestyle what is causing any particular problem, i.e. a lot of driving could lead to backache. You need detailed information about the client to treat them holistically.*

Treatment Plan

> **TIP** — *Here you can explain what the client would like you to help them with. For example, do they have a bad back? You would choose oils that help relieve aches and pains, or are antispasmodic. Will your plan be focusing on any particular area of the body?*

Treatment One

Refer to Lesson 10: Carrier Oils for determining which oils are best for certain conditions.

Details of How The Treatment Was Conducted

> **TIP** — *What methods were recommended in essential oil usage?*

Details of How The Client Felt Before, During and After The Treatment

> **TIP** — *Here you can point out the client's disposition, and/or any physical/emotional problems they have.*

Home Care and After Care Advice

TIP — *Note recommended methods for self-treatments i.e. baths, compresses, etc. with quantities of oil and frequency of use. Advise client of normal reactions to treatments — such as feeling tired, etc. Inform client of any aftereffects of oils i.e. phototoxic so stay out of the sun.*

Reflective Practice

TIP — *How did you perform as a therapist? Were you nervous/confident?*

Treatment Follow Up

TIP — *Check your consultation form for any changes since initial visit. Make sure that the client has not become pregnant, has had any bad reactions, or is on any new medications, etc.*

Overall Conclusion

TIP — *Did your recommendations accomplish their goals? Did you learn anything from treating this client? Would you have done anything differently?*

ACP-1 ACTIVITY: AROMATHERAPY CLIENT INTAKE FORM

In this course, we covered making aromatic and therapeutic blends for treating sicknesses and diseases. You will find most people are interested in finding answers to their health concerns and are seeking an alternative to prescribed medicines. As you have learned, therapeutic grade essential oils do offer us a great option to meds!

For those who would like to pursue a career in aromatherapy as a Certified Aromatherapist, performing a case study will give you an opportunity to start your practice. In this activity, you will use this intake form just like you would if you were practicing clinical aromatherapy.

Use this form to collect data for your client (this can be yourself or a friend). It is important to get as much health history as possible in guiding users on which essential oils will benefit them. With this information, write up a case study (using the 2nd form that follows) for a prescribed treatment plan using essential oils. Feel free to ad lib if you do not have a "health issue" or a friend willing to volunteer.

Aromatherapy Intake Form

First Name: _____ Last Name: _____

Date of Birth: _____ / _____ / _____

Address: _____

_____

City: _____ State: _____ Zip: _____

Phone Number: _____ Email: _____

1. *How would you describe your overall health?*

_____
_____
_____
_____
_____

2. What are you hoping essential oils can do for your health?
_____
_____
_____
_____

3. Do you have any chronic illnesses? If yes, what type of condition?
_____
_____
_____
_____

4. How long have you been aware of this condition?
_____
_____
_____
_____

5. What type of treatment(s) have you tried?
_____
_____
_____
_____

6. What has helped?
_____
_____
_____
_____

7. *What symptoms are most difficult for you?*

_____
_____
_____
_____

8. *Do you have any acute conditions you would like to address?*

_____
_____
_____
_____

9. *Please list any allergies:*

_____   _____
_____   _____
_____   _____

10. *Are you pregnant or trying to become pregnant?*   Yes ☐   No ☐

11. *Do you have epilepsy?*   Yes ☐   No ☐

12. *Do you have high/low blood pressure?*   Yes ☐   No ☐

13. *Which oils or aromas are you drawn to?*

_____   _____
_____   _____
_____   _____

14. *Do any oils or aromas disturb you?*

_____
_____
_____
_____

15. *Are you under the care of a physician? If so, please list the condition(s) you are being treated for:*

_____
_____
_____
_____

16. *Please list any medications you are taking:*

_____   _____
_____   _____
_____   _____

Since essential oils should not be used under certain circumstances, I affirm that I have truthfully answered all questions pertaining to my health on the Aromatherapy Intake Form. *Please sign below.*

Signature:_____

Date:_____ / _____ / _____

Aromatherapy Clinical Practice Intake Notes

For your aromatherapy clinical practice, you will need to make intake notes for each client.
Use this form as a guide to help you get started.

Client Profile & Lifestyle

TIP — *Here you can write a summary of what is covered in the consultation form. You should be able to see from the client's lifestyle what is causing any particular problem, i.e. a lot of driving could lead to backache. You need detailed information about the client to treat them holistically.*

Treatment Plan

TIP — *Here you can explain what the client would like you to help them with. For example, do they have a bad back? You would choose oils that help relieve aches and pains, or are antispasmodic. Will your plan be focusing on any particular area of the body?*

Treatment One

Refer to Lesson 10: Carrier Oils for determining which oils are best for certain conditions.

Details of How The Treatment Was Conducted

TIP — *What methods were recommended in essential oil usage?*

Details of How The Client Felt Before, During and After The Treatment

TIP — *Here you can point out the client's disposition, and/or any physical/emotional problems they have.*

Home Care and After Care Advice

TIP — *Note recommended methods for self-treatments i.e. baths, compresses, etc. with quantities of oil and frequency of use. Advise client of normal reactions to treatments — such as feeling tired, etc. Inform client of any aftereffects of oils i.e. phototoxic so stay out of the sun.*

Reflective Practice

TIP — *How did you perform as a therapist? Were you nervous/confident?*

Treatment Follow Up

TIP — *Check your consultation form for any changes since initial visit. Make sure that the client has not become pregnant, has had any bad reactions, or is on any new medications, etc.*

Overall Conclusion

TIP — *Did your recommendations accomplish their goals? Did you learn anything from treating this client? Would you have done anything differently?*

ACP-1 ACTIVITY: AROMATHERAPY CLIENT INTAKE FORM

In this course, we covered making aromatic and therapeutic blends for treating sicknesses and diseases. You will find most people are interested in finding answers to their health concerns and are seeking an alternative to prescribed medicines. As you have learned, therapeutic grade essential oils do offer us a great option to meds!

For those who would like to pursue a career in aromatherapy as a Certified Aromatherapist, performing a case study will give you an opportunity to start your practice. In this activity, you will use this intake form just like you would if you were practicing clinical aromatherapy.

Use this form to collect data for your client (this can be yourself or a friend). It is important to get as much health history as possible in guiding users on which essential oils will benefit them. With this information, write up a case study (using the 2nd form that follows) for a prescribed treatment plan using essential oils. Feel free to ad lib if you do not have a "health issue" or a friend willing to volunteer.

Aromatherapy Intake Form

First Name: _____ Last Name: _____

Date of Birth: _____ / _____ / _____

Address: _____
_____

City: _____ State: _____ Zip: _____

Phone Number: _____ Email: _____

1. *How would you describe your overall health?*

_____
_____
_____
_____
_____

2. What are you hoping essential oils can do for your health?

_____
_____
_____
_____

3. Do you have any chronic illnesses? If yes, what type of condition?

_____
_____
_____
_____

4. How long have you been aware of this condition?

_____
_____
_____
_____

5. What type of treatment(s) have you tried?

_____
_____
_____
_____

6. What has helped?

_____
_____
_____
_____

7. *What symptoms are most difficult for you?*

_____
_____
_____
_____

8. *Do you have any acute conditions you would like to address?*

_____
_____
_____
_____

9. *Please list any allergies:*

_____   _____
_____   _____
_____   _____

10. *Are you pregnant or trying to become pregnant?* Yes ☐   No ☐

11. *Do you have epilepsy?* Yes ☐   No ☐

12. *Do you have high/low blood pressure?* Yes ☐   No ☐

13. *Which oils or aromas are you drawn to?*

_____   _____
_____   _____
_____   _____

14. *Do any oils or aromas disturb you?*

_____
_____
_____
_____

15. *Are you under the care of a physician? If so, please list the condition(s) you are being treated for:*

_____
_____
_____
_____

16. *Please list any medications you are taking:*

_____   _____
_____   _____
_____   _____
_____   _____

Since essential oils should not be used under certain circumstances, I affirm that I have truthfully answered all questions pertaining to my health on the Aromatherapy Intake Form. *Please sign below.*

Signature:_____

Date: _____ / _____ / _____

Aromatherapy Clinical Practice Intake Notes

For your aromatherapy clinical practice, you will need to make intake notes for each client.
Use this form as a guide to help you get started.

Client Profile & Lifestyle

TIP — *Here you can write a summary of what is covered in the consultation form. You should be able to see from the client's lifestyle what is causing any particular problem, i.e. a lot of driving could lead to backache. You need detailed information about the client to treat them holistically.*

Treatment Plan

TIP — *Here you can explain what the client would like you to help them with. For example, do they have a bad back? You would choose oils that help relieve aches and pains, or are antispasmodic. Will your plan be focusing on any particular area of the body?*

Treatment One

Refer to Lesson 10: Carrier Oils for determining which oils are best for certain conditions.

Details of How The Treatment Was Conducted

TIP — *What methods were recommended in essential oil usage?*

Details of How The Client Felt Before, During and After The Treatment

TIP — *Here you can point out the client's disposition, and/or any physical/emotional problems they have.*

Home Care and After Care Advice

TIP — *Note recommended methods for self-treatments i.e. baths, compresses, etc. with quantities of oil and frequency of use. Advise client of normal reactions to treatments — such as feeling tired, etc. Inform client of any aftereffects of oils i.e. phototoxic so stay out of the sun.*

Reflective Practice

TIP — *How did you perform as a therapist? Were you nervous/confident?*

Treatment Follow Up

TIP — *Check your consultation form for any changes since initial visit. Make sure that the client has not become pregnant, has had any bad reactions, or is on any new medications, etc.*

Overall Conclusion

TIP — *Did your recommendations accomplish their goals? Did you learn anything from treating this client? Would you have done anything differently?*

ACP-1 ACTIVITY: AROMATHERAPY CLIENT INTAKE FORM

In this course, we covered making aromatic and therapeutic blends for treating sicknesses and diseases. You will find most people are interested in finding answers to their health concerns and are seeking an alternative to prescribed medicines. As you have learned, therapeutic grade essential oils do offer us a great option to meds!

For those who would like to pursue a career in aromatherapy as a Certified Aromatherapist, performing a case study will give you an opportunity to start your practice. In this activity, you will use this intake form just like you would if you were practicing clinical aromatherapy.

Use this form to collect data for your client (this can be yourself or a friend). It is important to get as much health history as possible in guiding users on which essential oils will benefit them. With this information, write up a case study (using the 2nd form that follows) for a prescribed treatment plan using essential oils. Feel free to ad lib if you do not have a "health issue" or a friend willing to volunteer.

Aromatherapy Intake Form

First Name: _____ Last Name: _____

Date of Birth: _____ / _____ / _____

Address: _____
_____

City: _____ State: _____ Zip: _____

Phone Number: _____ Email: _____

1. *How would you describe your overall health?*

_____
_____
_____
_____
_____

2. *What are you hoping essential oils can do for your health?*

_____
_____
_____
_____

3. *Do you have any chronic illnesses? If yes, what type of condition?*

_____
_____
_____
_____

4. *How long have you been aware of this condition?*

_____
_____
_____
_____

5. *What type of treatment(s) have you tried?*

_____
_____
_____
_____

6. *What has helped?*

_____
_____
_____
_____

7. *What symptoms are most difficult for you?*

_____
_____
_____
_____

8. *Do you have any acute conditions you would like to address?*

_____
_____
_____
_____

9. *Please list any allergies:*

_____   _____
_____   _____
_____   _____

10. *Are you pregnant or trying to become pregnant?*   Yes ☐   No ☐

11. *Do you have epilepsy?*   Yes ☐   No ☐

12. *Do you have high/low blood pressure?*   Yes ☐   No ☐

13. *Which oils or aromas are you drawn to?*

_____   _____
_____   _____
_____   _____
_____   _____

14. *Do any oils or aromas disturb you?*

_____
_____
_____
_____

15. *Are you under the care of a physician? If so, please list the condition(s) you are being treated for:*

_____
_____
_____
_____

16. *Please list any medications you are taking:*

_____   _____
_____   _____
_____   _____
_____   _____

Since essential oils should not be used under certain circumstances, I affirm that I have truthfully answered all questions pertaining to my health on the Aromatherapy Intake Form. *Please sign below.*

Signature:_____

Date:_____ / _____ / _____

Aromatherapy Clinical Practice Intake Notes

For your aromatherapy clinical practice, you will need to make intake notes for each client.
Use this form as a guide to help you get started.

Client Profile & Lifestyle

TIP — *Here you can write a summary of what is covered in the consultation form. You should be able to see from the client's lifestyle what is causing any particular problem, i.e. a lot of driving could lead to backache. You need detailed information about the client to treat them holistically.*

Treatment Plan

TIP — *Here you can explain what the client would like you to help them with. For example, do they have a bad back? You would choose oils that help relieve aches and pains, or are antispasmodic. Will your plan be focusing on any particular area of the body?*

Treatment One

Refer to Lesson 10: Carrier Oils for determining which oils are best for certain conditions.

Details of How The Treatment Was Conducted

TIP — *What methods were recommended in essential oil usage?*

Details of How The Client Felt Before, During and After The Treatment

TIP — *Here you can point out the client's disposition, and/or any physical/emotional problems they have.*

Home Care and After Care Advice

TIP — *Note recommended methods for self-treatments i.e. baths, compresses, etc. with quantities of oil and frequency of use. Advise client of normal reactions to treatments — such as feeling tired, etc. Inform client of any aftereffects of oils i.e. phototoxic so stay out of the sun.*

Reflective Practice

TIP — *How did you perform as a therapist? Were you nervous/confident?*

Treatment Follow Up

TIP — *Check your consultation form for any changes since initial visit. Make sure that the client has not become pregnant, has had any bad reactions, or is on any new medications, etc.*

Overall Conclusion

TIP — *Did your recommendations accomplish their goals? Did you learn anything from treating this client? Would you have done anything differently?*

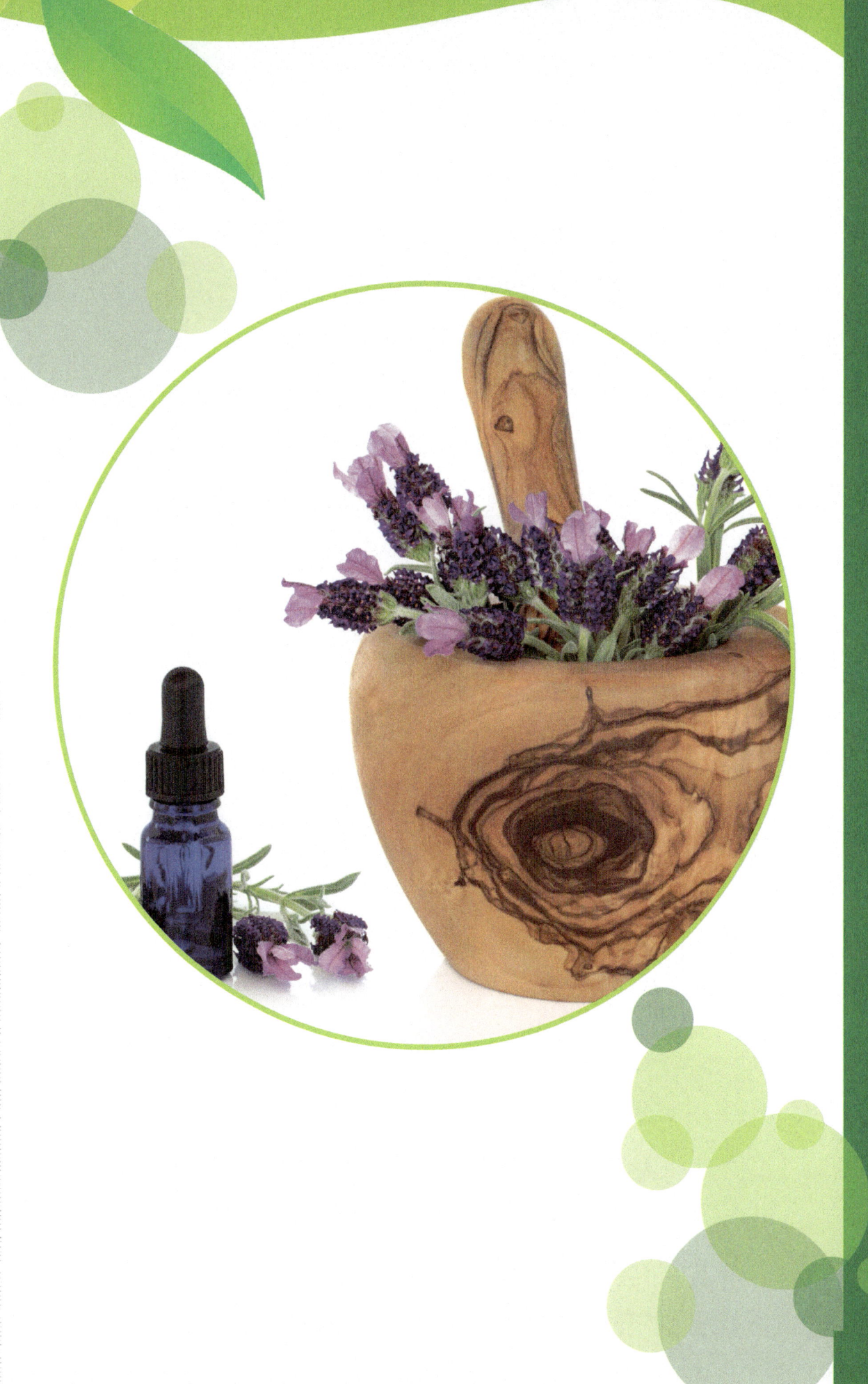

APOTHECARY NOTES

ACP-1 ACTIVITY: APOTHECARY NOTES

As you begin your aromatherapy practice, you will want to consider both the art and the science of aromatic and therapeutic blending when creating your formulation. Answer the following questions based on your evaluation of your client's specific needs. Use this information as a guide in determining what type of product you will make and which oils you will use to formulate your blend.

Client's Name: _____

1. What is the purpose of your blend? What are the results you hope to accomplish with your blend?

_____
_____
_____

2. Is it for aromatic or therapeutic benefits? _____

3. What kind of effect are you hoping to accomplish with this blend? Are you making it to help reduce swelling or alleviate pain, or is it to help bring a sense of calm to reduce anxiety and/or stress? Will it be stimulating or soothing? Look at how it will affect the whole person: body, mind and spirit.

_____
_____
_____

4. How will the blend be used? Will it be used as a room spray, in the bath, on the body with a lotion or carrier oil, as a massage oil, or placed in a diffuser for inhalation, etc.?

_____
_____
_____

5. Will this blend be used on an elderly person or young child? Note the person's age and gender (male or female). This will be important to know when determining the dilution rate.

_____
_____
_____

6. *How long will the blend be used? Is it for an acute treatment, illness or health condition? Determine the frequency (how many times a day to use it) and duration (how many days) for your blend.*

_____
_____
_____
_____

7. *How should your client use this blend? (For general purposes, a blend can be applied 6 times a day for acute conditions and 3-6 times a day for chronic complaints, or as needed.)*

_____
_____

8. *Is your blend for an acute treatment or condition? Determine and note whether it is for a viral, bacterial, fungal, or another type of infection. This will be pivotal in determining which essential oils to use.*

_____
_____
_____
_____

9. *Are there any contraindications or precautions you need to take into consideration as you make your blend? Be sure to check which oils are safe for any pre-existing health conditions that may exist.*

_____
_____

10. *What is the appropriate dosage of oils for this application? For instance, 15-18 drops of essential oil blend per 30 ml (one ounce) of carrier oil, applied 3-6 times a day (or as needed).*

_____
_____

ACP-1 ACTIVITY: APOTHECARY NOTES

As you begin your aromatherapy practice, you will want to consider both the art and the science of aromatic and therapeutic blending when creating your formulation. Answer the following questions based on your evaluation of your client's specific needs. Use this information as a guide in determining what type of product you will make and which oils you will use to formulate your blend.

Client's Name: _____

1. *What is the purpose of your blend? What are the results you hope to accomplish with your blend?*

_____
_____
_____

2. *Is it for aromatic or therapeutic benefits?* _____

3. *What kind of effect are you hoping to accomplish with this blend? Are you making it to help reduce swelling or alleviate pain, or is it to help bring a sense of calm to reduce anxiety and/or stress? Will it be stimulating or soothing? Look at how it will affect the whole person: body, mind and spirit.*

_____
_____
_____

4. *How will the blend be used? Will it be used as a room spray, in the bath, on the body with a lotion or carrier oil, as a massage oil, or placed in a diffuser for inhalation, etc.?*

_____
_____
_____

5. *Will this blend be used on an elderly person or young child? Note the person's age and gender (male or female). This will be important to know when determining the dilution rate.*

_____
_____
_____

6. *How long will the blend be used? Is it for an acute treatment, illness or health condition? Determine the frequency (how many times a day to use it) and duration (how many days) for your blend.*

_____
_____
_____
_____

7. *How should your client use this blend? (For general purposes, a blend can be applied 6 times a day for acute conditions and 3-6 times a day for chronic complaints, or as needed.)*

_____
_____

8. *Is your blend for an acute treatment or condition? Determine and note whether it is for a viral, bacterial, fungal, or another type of infection. This will be pivotal in determining which essential oils to use.*

_____
_____
_____
_____

9. *Are there any contraindications or precautions you need to take into consideration as you make your blend? Be sure to check which oils are safe for any pre-existing health conditions that may exist.*

_____
_____

10. *What is the appropriate dosage of oils for this application? For instance, 15-18 drops of essential oil blend per 30 ml (one ounce) of carrier oil, applied 3-6 times a day (or as needed).*

_____
_____

ACP-1 ACTIVITY: APOTHECARY NOTES

As you begin your aromatherapy practice, you will want to consider both the art and the science of aromatic and therapeutic blending when creating your formulation. Answer the following questions based on your evaluation of your client's specific needs. Use this information as a guide in determining what type of product you will make and which oils you will use to formulate your blend.

Client's Name: _____

1. *What is the purpose of your blend? What are the results you hope to accomplish with your blend?*

_____
_____
_____
_____

2. *Is it for aromatic or therapeutic benefits?* _____

3. *What kind of effect are you hoping to accomplish with this blend? Are you making it to help reduce swelling or alleviate pain, or is it to help bring a sense of calm to reduce anxiety and/or stress? Will it be stimulating or soothing? Look at how it will affect the whole person: body, mind and spirit.*

_____
_____
_____

4. *How will the blend be used? Will it be used as a room spray, in the bath, on the body with a lotion or carrier oil, as a massage oil, or placed in a diffuser for inhalation, etc.?*

_____
_____
_____

5. *Will this blend be used on an elderly person or young child? Note the person's age and gender (male or female). This will be important to know when determining the dilution rate.*

_____
_____
_____

6. *How long will the blend be used? Is it for an acute treatment, illness or health condition? Determine the frequency (how many times a day to use it) and duration (how many days) for your blend.*

_____
_____
_____
_____

7. *How should your client use this blend? (For general purposes, a blend can be applied 6 times a day for acute conditions and 3-6 times a day for chronic complaints, or as needed.)*

_____
_____

8. *Is your blend for an acute treatment or condition? Determine and note whether it is for a viral, bacterial, fungal, or another type of infection. This will be pivotal in determining which essential oils to use.*

_____
_____
_____
_____

9. *Are there any contraindications or precautions you need to take into consideration as you make your blend? Be sure to check which oils are safe for any pre-existing health conditions that may exist.*

_____
_____

10. *What is the appropriate dosage of oils for this application? For instance, 15-18 drops of essential oil blend per 30 ml (one ounce) of carrier oil, applied 3-6 times a day (or as needed).*

_____
_____

ACP-1 ACTIVITY: APOTHECARY NOTES

As you begin your aromatherapy practice, you will want to consider both the art and the science of aromatic and therapeutic blending when creating your formulation. Answer the following questions based on your evaluation of your client's specific needs. Use this information as a guide in determining what type of product you will make and which oils you will use to formulate your blend.

Client's Name: _____

1. What is the purpose of your blend? What are the results you hope to accomplish with your blend?

_____
_____
_____

2. Is it for aromatic or therapeutic benefits? _____

3. What kind of effect are you hoping to accomplish with this blend? Are you making it to help reduce swelling or alleviate pain, or is it to help bring a sense of calm to reduce anxiety and/or stress? Will it be stimulating or soothing? Look at how it will affect the whole person: body, mind and spirit.

_____
_____
_____

4. How will the blend be used? Will it be used as a room spray, in the bath, on the body with a lotion or carrier oil, as a massage oil, or placed in a diffuser for inhalation, etc.?

_____
_____
_____

5. Will this blend be used on an elderly person or young child? Note the person's age and gender (male or female). This will be important to know when determining the dilution rate.

_____
_____
_____

6. *How long will the blend be used? Is it for an acute treatment, illness or health condition? Determine the frequency (how many times a day to use it) and duration (how many days) for your blend.*

_____

_____

_____

_____

7. *How should your client use this blend? (For general purposes, a blend can be applied 6 times a day for acute conditions and 3-6 times a day for chronic complaints, or as needed.)*

_____

_____

8. *Is your blend for an acute treatment or condition? Determine and note whether it is for a viral, bacterial, fungal, or another type of infection. This will be pivotal in determining which essential oils to use.*

_____

_____

_____

_____

9. *Are there any contraindications or precautions you need to take into consideration as you make your blend? Be sure to check which oils are safe for any pre-existing health conditions that may exist.*

_____

_____

10. *What is the appropriate dosage of oils for this application? For instance, 15-18 drops of essential oil blend per 30 ml (one ounce) of carrier oil, applied 3-6 times a day (or as needed).*

_____

_____

ACP-1 ACTIVITY: APOTHECARY NOTES

As you begin your aromatherapy practice, you will want to consider both the art and the science of aromatic and therapeutic blending when creating your formulation. Answer the following questions based on your evaluation of your client's specific needs. Use this information as a guide in determining what type of product you will make and which oils you will use to formulate your blend.

Client's Name: _____

1. *What is the purpose of your blend? What are the results you hope to accomplish with your blend?*

_____
_____
_____

2. *Is it for aromatic or therapeutic benefits?* _____

3. *What kind of effect are you hoping to accomplish with this blend? Are you making it to help reduce swelling or alleviate pain, or is it to help bring a sense of calm to reduce anxiety and/or stress? Will it be stimulating or soothing? Look at how it will affect the whole person: body, mind and spirit.*

_____
_____
_____

4. *How will the blend be used? Will it be used as a room spray, in the bath, on the body with a lotion or carrier oil, as a massage oil, or placed in a diffuser for inhalation, etc.?*

_____
_____
_____

5. *Will this blend be used on an elderly person or young child? Note the person's age and gender (male or female). This will be important to know when determining the dilution rate.*

_____
_____

6. *How long will the blend be used? Is it for an acute treatment, illness or health condition? Determine the frequency (how many times a day to use it) and duration (how many days) for your blend.*

_____
_____
_____
_____

7. *How should your client use this blend? (For general purposes, a blend can be applied 6 times a day for acute conditions and 3-6 times a day for chronic complaints, or as needed.)*

_____
_____

8. *Is your blend for an acute treatment or condition? Determine and note whether it is for a viral, bacterial, fungal, or another type of infection. This will be pivotal in determining which essential oils to use.*

_____
_____
_____
_____

9. *Are there any contraindications or precautions you need to take into consideration as you make your blend? Be sure to check which oils are safe for any pre-existing health conditions that may exist.*

_____
_____

10. *What is the appropriate dosage of oils for this application? For instance, 15-18 drops of essential oil blend per 30 ml (one ounce) of carrier oil, applied 3-6 times a day (or as needed).*

_____
_____

ACP-1 ACTIVITY: APOTHECARY NOTES

As you begin your aromatherapy practice, you will want to consider both the art and the science of aromatic and therapeutic blending when creating your formulation. Answer the following questions based on your evaluation of your client's specific needs. Use this information as a guide in determining what type of product you will make and which oils you will use to formulate your blend.

Client's Name: _____

1. *What is the purpose of your blend? What are the results you hope to accomplish with your blend?*

   _____
   _____
   _____
   _____

2. *Is it for aromatic or therapeutic benefits?* _____

3. *What kind of effect are you hoping to accomplish with this blend? Are you making it to help reduce swelling or alleviate pain, or is it to help bring a sense of calm to reduce anxiety and/or stress? Will it be stimulating or soothing? Look at how it will affect the whole person: body, mind and spirit.*

   _____
   _____
   _____
   _____

4. *How will the blend be used? Will it be used as a room spray, in the bath, on the body with a lotion or carrier oil, as a massage oil, or placed in a diffuser for inhalation, etc.?*

   _____
   _____
   _____
   _____

5. *Will this blend be used on an elderly person or young child? Note the person's age and gender (male or female). This will be important to know when determining the dilution rate.*

   _____
   _____
   _____
   _____

6. *How long will the blend be used? Is it for an acute treatment, illness or health condition? Determine the frequency (how many times a day to use it) and duration (how many days) for your blend.*

_____

_____

_____

_____

7. *How should your client use this blend? (For general purposes, a blend can be applied 6 times a day for acute conditions and 3-6 times a day for chronic complaints, or as needed.)*

_____

_____

8. *Is your blend for an acute treatment or condition? Determine and note whether it is for a viral, bacterial, fungal, or another type of infection. This will be pivotal in determining which essential oils to use.*

_____

_____

_____

_____

9. *Are there any contraindications or precautions you need to take into consideration as you make your blend? Be sure to check which oils are safe for any pre-existing health conditions that may exist.*

_____

_____

10. *What is the appropriate dosage of oils for this application? For instance, 15-18 drops of essential oil blend per 30 ml (one ounce) of carrier oil, applied 3-6 times a day (or as needed).*

_____

_____

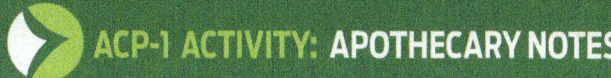

ACP-1 ACTIVITY: APOTHECARY NOTES

As you begin your aromatherapy practice, you will want to consider both the art and the science of aromatic and therapeutic blending when creating your formulation. Answer the following questions based on your evaluation of your client's specific needs. Use this information as a guide in determining what type of product you will make and which oils you will use to formulate your blend.

Client's Name: _____

1. *What is the purpose of your blend? What are the results you hope to accomplish with your blend?*

_____
_____
_____

2. *Is it for aromatic or therapeutic benefits?* _____

3. *What kind of effect are you hoping to accomplish with this blend? Are you making it to help reduce swelling or alleviate pain, or is it to help bring a sense of calm to reduce anxiety and/or stress? Will it be stimulating or soothing? Look at how it will affect the whole person: body, mind and spirit.*

_____
_____
_____

4. *How will the blend be used? Will it be used as a room spray, in the bath, on the body with a lotion or carrier oil, as a massage oil, or placed in a diffuser for inhalation, etc.?*

_____
_____
_____

5. *Will this blend be used on an elderly person or young child? Note the person's age and gender (male or female). This will be important to know when determining the dilution rate.*

_____
_____
_____

6. *How long will the blend be used? Is it for an acute treatment, illness or health condition? Determine the frequency (how many times a day to use it) and duration (how many days) for your blend.*

_____

_____

_____

7. *How should your client use this blend? (For general purposes, a blend can be applied 6 times a day for acute conditions and 3-6 times a day for chronic complaints, or as needed.)*

_____

_____

8. *Is your blend for an acute treatment or condition? Determine and note whether it is for a viral, bacterial, fungal, or another type of infection. This will be pivotal in determining which essential oils to use.*

_____

_____

_____

9. *Are there any contraindications or precautions you need to take into consideration as you make your blend? Be sure to check which oils are safe for any pre-existing health conditions that may exist.*

_____

_____

10. *What is the appropriate dosage of oils for this application? For instance, 15-18 drops of essential oil blend per 30 ml (one ounce) of carrier oil, applied 3-6 times a day (or as needed).*

_____

_____

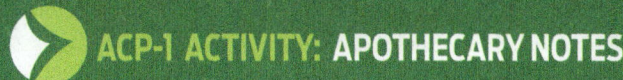

ACP-1 ACTIVITY: APOTHECARY NOTES

As you begin your aromatherapy practice, you will want to consider both the art and the science of aromatic and therapeutic blending when creating your formulation. Answer the following questions based on your evaluation of your client's specific needs. Use this information as a guide in determining what type of product you will make and which oils you will use to formulate your blend.

Client's Name: _____

1. What is the purpose of your blend? What are the results you hope to accomplish with your blend?

_____
_____
_____

2. Is it for aromatic or therapeutic benefits? _____

3. What kind of effect are you hoping to accomplish with this blend? Are you making it to help reduce swelling or alleviate pain, or is it to help bring a sense of calm to reduce anxiety and/or stress? Will it be stimulating or soothing? Look at how it will affect the whole person: body, mind and spirit.

_____
_____
_____

4. How will the blend be used? Will it be used as a room spray, in the bath, on the body with a lotion or carrier oil, as a massage oil, or placed in a diffuser for inhalation, etc.?

_____
_____
_____

5. Will this blend be used on an elderly person or young child? Note the person's age and gender (male or female). This will be important to know when determining the dilution rate.

_____
_____

6. *How long will the blend be used? Is it for an acute treatment, illness or health condition? Determine the frequency (how many times a day to use it) and duration (how many days) for your blend.*

_____
_____
_____
_____

7. *How should your client use this blend? (For general purposes, a blend can be applied 6 times a day for acute conditions and 3-6 times a day for chronic complaints, or as needed.)*

_____
_____

8. *Is your blend for an acute treatment or condition? Determine and note whether it is for a viral, bacterial, fungal, or another type of infection. This will be pivotal in determining which essential oils to use.*

_____
_____
_____
_____

9. *Are there any contraindications or precautions you need to take into consideration as you make your blend? Be sure to check which oils are safe for any pre-existing health conditions that may exist.*

_____
_____

10. *What is the appropriate dosage of oils for this application? For instance, 15-18 drops of essential oil blend per 30 ml (one ounce) of carrier oil, applied 3-6 times a day (or as needed).*

_____
_____

ACP-1 ACTIVITY: APOTHECARY NOTES

As you begin your aromatherapy practice, you will want to consider both the art and the science of aromatic and therapeutic blending when creating your formulation. Answer the following questions based on your evaluation of your client's specific needs. Use this information as a guide in determining what type of product you will make and which oils you will use to formulate your blend.

Client's Name: _____

1. *What is the purpose of your blend? What are the results you hope to accomplish with your blend?*

   _____
   _____
   _____
   _____

2. *Is it for aromatic or therapeutic benefits?* _____

3. *What kind of effect are you hoping to accomplish with this blend? Are you making it to help reduce swelling or alleviate pain, or is it to help bring a sense of calm to reduce anxiety and/or stress? Will it be stimulating or soothing? Look at how it will affect the whole person: body, mind and spirit.*

   _____
   _____
   _____
   _____

4. *How will the blend be used? Will it be used as a room spray, in the bath, on the body with a lotion or carrier oil, as a massage oil, or placed in a diffuser for inhalation, etc.?*

   _____
   _____
   _____
   _____

5. *Will this blend be used on an elderly person or young child? Note the person's age and gender (male or female). This will be important to know when determining the dilution rate.*

   _____
   _____
   _____

6. *How long will the blend be used? Is it for an acute treatment, illness or health condition? Determine the frequency (how many times a day to use it) and duration (how many days) for your blend.*

_____
_____
_____
_____

7. *How should your client use this blend? (For general purposes, a blend can be applied 6 times a day for acute conditions and 3-6 times a day for chronic complaints, or as needed.)*

_____
_____

8. *Is your blend for an acute treatment or condition? Determine and note whether it is for a viral, bacterial, fungal, or another type of infection. This will be pivotal in determining which essential oils to use.*

_____
_____
_____
_____

9. *Are there any contraindications or precautions you need to take into consideration as you make your blend? Be sure to check which oils are safe for any pre-existing health conditions that may exist.*

_____
_____

10. *What is the appropriate dosage of oils for this application? For instance, 15-18 drops of essential oil blend per 30 ml (one ounce) of carrier oil, applied 3-6 times a day (or as needed).*

_____
_____

ACP-1 ACTIVITY: APOTHECARY NOTES

As you begin your aromatherapy practice, you will want to consider both the art and the science of aromatic and therapeutic blending when creating your formulation. Answer the following questions based on your evaluation of your client's specific needs. Use this information as a guide in determining what type of product you will make and which oils you will use to formulate your blend.

Client's Name: _____

1. *What is the purpose of your blend? What are the results you hope to accomplish with your blend?*

_____
_____
_____

2. *Is it for aromatic or therapeutic benefits?* _____

3. *What kind of effect are you hoping to accomplish with this blend? Are you making it to help reduce swelling or alleviate pain, or is it to help bring a sense of calm to reduce anxiety and/or stress? Will it be stimulating or soothing? Look at how it will affect the whole person: body, mind and spirit.*

_____
_____
_____

4. *How will the blend be used? Will it be used as a room spray, in the bath, on the body with a lotion or carrier oil, as a massage oil, or placed in a diffuser for inhalation, etc.?*

_____
_____
_____

5. *Will this blend be used on an elderly person or young child? Note the person's age and gender (male or female). This will be important to know when determining the dilution rate.*

_____
_____
_____

6. *How long will the blend be used? Is it for an acute treatment, illness or health condition? Determine the frequency (how many times a day to use it) and duration (how many days) for your blend.*

_____

_____

_____

_____

7. *How should your client use this blend? (For general purposes, a blend can be applied 6 times a day for acute conditions and 3-6 times a day for chronic complaints, or as needed.)*

_____

_____

8. *Is your blend for an acute treatment or condition? Determine and note whether it is for a viral, bacterial, fungal, or another type of infection. This will be pivotal in determining which essential oils to use.*

_____

_____

_____

_____

9. *Are there any contraindications or precautions you need to take into consideration as you make your blend? Be sure to check which oils are safe for any pre-existing health conditions that may exist.*

_____

_____

10. *What is the appropriate dosage of oils for this application? For instance, 15-18 drops of essential oil blend per 30 ml (one ounce) of carrier oil, applied 3-6 times a day (or as needed).*

_____

_____

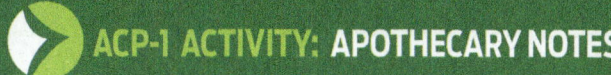

ACP-1 ACTIVITY: APOTHECARY NOTES

As you begin your aromatherapy practice, you will want to consider both the art and the science of aromatic and therapeutic blending when creating your formulation. Answer the following questions based on your evaluation of your client's specific needs. Use this information as a guide in determining what type of product you will make and which oils you will use to formulate your blend.

Client's Name: _____

1. *What is the purpose of your blend? What are the results you hope to accomplish with your blend?*

_____
_____
_____
_____

2. *Is it for aromatic or therapeutic benefits?* _____

3. *What kind of effect are you hoping to accomplish with this blend? Are you making it to help reduce swelling or alleviate pain, or is it to help bring a sense of calm to reduce anxiety and/or stress? Will it be stimulating or soothing? Look at how it will affect the whole person: body, mind and spirit.*

_____
_____
_____

4. *How will the blend be used? Will it be used as a room spray, in the bath, on the body with a lotion or carrier oil, as a massage oil, or placed in a diffuser for inhalation, etc.?*

_____
_____
_____

5. *Will this blend be used on an elderly person or young child? Note the person's age and gender (male or female). This will be important to know when determining the dilution rate.*

_____
_____
_____

6. *How long will the blend be used? Is it for an acute treatment, illness or health condition? Determine the frequency (how many times a day to use it) and duration (how many days) for your blend.*

_____
_____
_____
_____

7. *How should your client use this blend? (For general purposes, a blend can be applied 6 times a day for acute conditions and 3-6 times a day for chronic complaints, or as needed.)*

_____
_____

8. *Is your blend for an acute treatment or condition? Determine and note whether it is for a viral, bacterial, fungal, or another type of infection. This will be pivotal in determining which essential oils to use.*

_____
_____
_____
_____

9. *Are there any contraindications or precautions you need to take into consideration as you make your blend? Be sure to check which oils are safe for any pre-existing health conditions that may exist.*

_____
_____

10. *What is the appropriate dosage of oils for this application? For instance, 15-18 drops of essential oil blend per 30 ml (one ounce) of carrier oil, applied 3-6 times a day (or as needed).*

_____
_____

ACP-1 ACTIVITY: APOTHECARY NOTES

As you begin your aromatherapy practice, you will want to consider both the art and the science of aromatic and therapeutic blending when creating your formulation. Answer the following questions based on your evaluation of your client's specific needs. Use this information as a guide in determining what type of product you will make and which oils you will use to formulate your blend.

Client's Name: _____

1. *What is the purpose of your blend? What are the results you hope to accomplish with your blend?*

   _____
   _____
   _____

2. *Is it for aromatic or therapeutic benefits?* _____

3. *What kind of effect are you hoping to accomplish with this blend? Are you making it to help reduce swelling or alleviate pain, or is it to help bring a sense of calm to reduce anxiety and/or stress? Will it be stimulating or soothing? Look at how it will affect the whole person: body, mind and spirit.*

   _____
   _____
   _____

4. *How will the blend be used? Will it be used as a room spray, in the bath, on the body with a lotion or carrier oil, as a massage oil, or placed in a diffuser for inhalation, etc.?*

   _____
   _____
   _____

5. *Will this blend be used on an elderly person or young child? Note the person's age and gender (male or female). This will be important to know when determining the dilution rate.*

   _____
   _____
   _____

6. *How long will the blend be used? Is it for an acute treatment, illness or health condition? Determine the frequency (how many times a day to use it) and duration (how many days) for your blend.*

_____

_____

_____

_____

7. *How should your client use this blend? (For general purposes, a blend can be applied 6 times a day for acute conditions and 3-6 times a day for chronic complaints, or as needed.)*

_____

_____

8. *Is your blend for an acute treatment or condition? Determine and note whether it is for a viral, bacterial, fungal, or another type of infection. This will be pivotal in determining which essential oils to use.*

_____

_____

_____

_____

9. *Are there any contraindications or precautions you need to take into consideration as you make your blend? Be sure to check which oils are safe for any pre-existing health conditions that may exist.*

_____

_____

10. *What is the appropriate dosage of oils for this application? For instance, 15-18 drops of essential oil blend per 30 ml (one ounce) of carrier oil, applied 3-6 times a day (or as needed).*

_____

_____

ACP-1 ACTIVITY: APOTHECARY NOTES

As you begin your aromatherapy practice, you will want to consider both the art and the science of aromatic and therapeutic blending when creating your formulation. Answer the following questions based on your evaluation of your client's specific needs. Use this information as a guide in determining what type of product you will make and which oils you will use to formulate your blend.

Client's Name: _____

1. *What is the purpose of your blend? What are the results you hope to accomplish with your blend?*

_____
_____
_____

2. *Is it for aromatic or therapeutic benefits?* _____

3. *What kind of effect are you hoping to accomplish with this blend? Are you making it to help reduce swelling or alleviate pain, or is it to help bring a sense of calm to reduce anxiety and/or stress? Will it be stimulating or soothing? Look at how it will affect the whole person: body, mind and spirit.*

_____
_____
_____

4. *How will the blend be used? Will it be used as a room spray, in the bath, on the body with a lotion or carrier oil, as a massage oil, or placed in a diffuser for inhalation, etc.?*

_____
_____
_____

5. *Will this blend be used on an elderly person or young child? Note the person's age and gender (male or female). This will be important to know when determining the dilution rate.*

_____
_____
_____

6. *How long will the blend be used? Is it for an acute treatment, illness or health condition? Determine the frequency (how many times a day to use it) and duration (how many days) for your blend.*

_____

_____

_____

_____

7. *How should your client use this blend? (For general purposes, a blend can be applied 6 times a day for acute conditions and 3-6 times a day for chronic complaints, or as needed.)*

_____

_____

8. *Is your blend for an acute treatment or condition? Determine and note whether it is for a viral, bacterial, fungal, or another type of infection. This will be pivotal in determining which essential oils to use.*

_____

_____

_____

_____

9. *Are there any contraindications or precautions you need to take into consideration as you make your blend? Be sure to check which oils are safe for any pre-existing health conditions that may exist.*

_____

_____

10. *What is the appropriate dosage of oils for this application? For instance, 15-18 drops of essential oil blend per 30 ml (one ounce) of carrier oil, applied 3-6 times a day (or as needed).*

_____

_____

ACP-1 ACTIVITY: APOTHECARY NOTES

As you begin your aromatherapy practice, you will want to consider both the art and the science of aromatic and therapeutic blending when creating your formulation. Answer the following questions based on your evaluation of your client's specific needs. Use this information as a guide in determining what type of product you will make and which oils you will use to formulate your blend.

Client's Name: _____

1. *What is the purpose of your blend? What are the results you hope to accomplish with your blend?*

   _____
   _____
   _____

2. *Is it for aromatic or therapeutic benefits?* _____

3. *What kind of effect are you hoping to accomplish with this blend? Are you making it to help reduce swelling or alleviate pain, or is it to help bring a sense of calm to reduce anxiety and/or stress? Will it be stimulating or soothing? Look at how it will affect the whole person: body, mind and spirit.*

   _____
   _____
   _____

4. *How will the blend be used? Will it be used as a room spray, in the bath, on the body with a lotion or carrier oil, as a massage oil, or placed in a diffuser for inhalation, etc.?*

   _____
   _____
   _____

5. *Will this blend be used on an elderly person or young child? Note the person's age and gender (male or female). This will be important to know when determining the dilution rate.*

   _____
   _____
   _____

6. *How long will the blend be used? Is it for an acute treatment, illness or health condition? Determine the frequency (how many times a day to use it) and duration (how many days) for your blend.*

_____
_____
_____
_____

7. *How should your client use this blend? (For general purposes, a blend can be applied 6 times a day for acute conditions and 3-6 times a day for chronic complaints, or as needed.)*

_____
_____
_____

8. *Is your blend for an acute treatment or condition? Determine and note whether it is for a viral, bacterial, fungal, or another type of infection. This will be pivotal in determining which essential oils to use.*

_____
_____
_____
_____

9. *Are there any contraindications or precautions you need to take into consideration as you make your blend? Be sure to check which oils are safe for any pre-existing health conditions that may exist.*

_____
_____

10. *What is the appropriate dosage of oils for this application? For instance, 15-18 drops of essential oil blend per 30 ml (one ounce) of carrier oil, applied 3-6 times a day (or as needed).*

_____
_____

ACP-1 ACTIVITY: APOTHECARY NOTES

As you begin your aromatherapy practice, you will want to consider both the art and the science of aromatic and therapeutic blending when creating your formulation. Answer the following questions based on your evaluation of your client's specific needs. Use this information as a guide in determining what type of product you will make and which oils you will use to formulate your blend.

Client's Name: _____

1. *What is the purpose of your blend? What are the results you hope to accomplish with your blend?*

   _____
   _____
   _____

2. *Is it for aromatic or therapeutic benefits?* _____

3. *What kind of effect are you hoping to accomplish with this blend? Are you making it to help reduce swelling or alleviate pain, or is it to help bring a sense of calm to reduce anxiety and/or stress? Will it be stimulating or soothing? Look at how it will affect the whole person: body, mind and spirit.*

   _____
   _____
   _____

4. *How will the blend be used? Will it be used as a room spray, in the bath, on the body with a lotion or carrier oil, as a massage oil, or placed in a diffuser for inhalation, etc.?*

   _____
   _____
   _____

5. *Will this blend be used on an elderly person or young child? Note the person's age and gender (male or female). This will be important to know when determining the dilution rate.*

   _____
   _____
   _____

6. *How long will the blend be used? Is it for an acute treatment, illness or health condition? Determine the frequency (how many times a day to use it) and duration (how many days) for your blend.*

_____
_____
_____
_____

7. *How should your client use this blend? (For general purposes, a blend can be applied 6 times a day for acute conditions and 3-6 times a day for chronic complaints, or as needed.)*

_____
_____

8. *Is your blend for an acute treatment or condition? Determine and note whether it is for a viral, bacterial, fungal, or another type of infection. This will be pivotal in determining which essential oils to use.*

_____
_____
_____
_____

9. *Are there any contraindications or precautions you need to take into consideration as you make your blend? Be sure to check which oils are safe for any pre-existing health conditions that may exist.*

_____
_____

10. *What is the appropriate dosage of oils for this application? For instance, 15-18 drops of essential oil blend per 30 ml (one ounce) of carrier oil, applied 3-6 times a day (or as needed).*

_____
_____

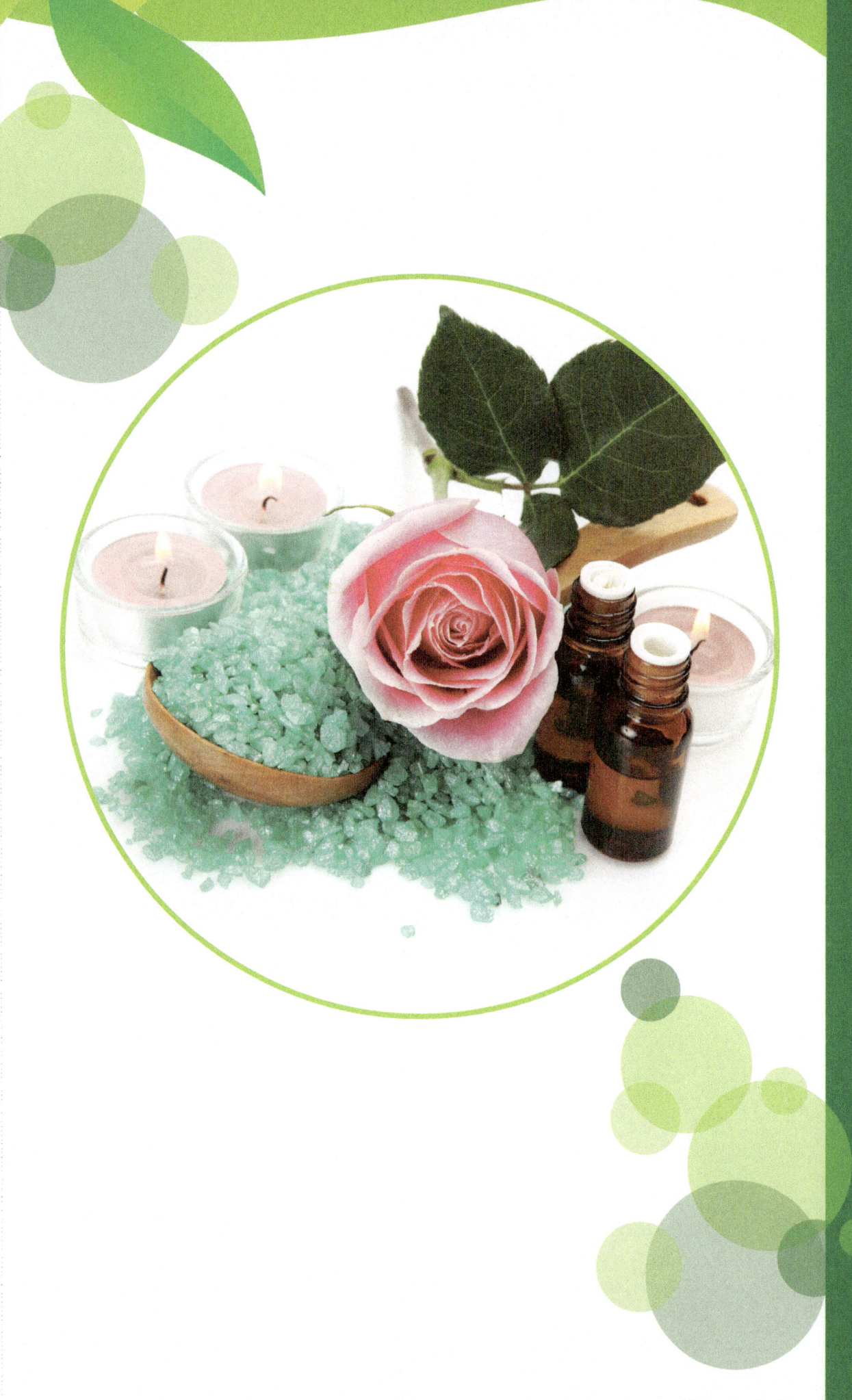

ESSENTIAL OIL DATASHEET FORMS

ESSENTIAL OIL DATASHEET FORM

Use this form to create your own datasheets for essential oils you have in your collection. You will need to do some research online or from books on hand to gather the information regarding your particular oil.

Oil Name: _____

Brief Description: _____
_____
_____

- **Country of Origin:** _____
- **Extraction Method:** _____
- **Plant Parts:** _____
- **Botanical Family:** _____
- **Chemical Families:** _____
- **Aroma:** _____
- **Note:** _____

PRECAUTIONS _____

Therapeutic Properties

USES

Bones/Joints: _____
_____

Circulatory: _____
_____

Digestive: _____
_____

Immune: _____
_____

Lymphatic: _____
_____

Mental/Emotional: _____
_____

Muscular/Joint: _____
_____

Reproductive: _____
_____

Respiratory: _____
_____

Skin: _____
_____

Urinary: _____
_____

SAFETY

_____
_____
_____

ESSENTIAL OIL DATASHEET FORM

Use this form to create your own datasheets for essential oils you have in your collection. You will need to do some research online or from books on hand to gather the information regarding your particular oil.

Oil Name: _____

Brief Description: _____
_____
_____

- Country of Origin: _____
- Extraction Method: _____
- Plant Parts: _____
- Botanical Family: _____
- Chemical Families: _____
- Aroma: _____
- Note: _____

PRECAUTIONS _____

Therapeutic Properties

USES

Bones/Joints: _____
_____

Circulatory: _____
_____

Digestive: _____
_____

Immune: _____
_____

Lymphatic: _____
_____

Mental/Emotional: _____
_____

Muscular/Joint: _____
_____

Reproductive: _____
_____

Respiratory: _____
_____

Skin: _____
_____

Urinary: _____
_____

SAFETY

_____
_____
_____

ESSENTIAL OIL DATASHEET FORM

Use this form to create your own datasheets for essential oils you have in your collection. You will need to do some research online or from books on hand to gather the information regarding your particular oil.

Oil Name: _____

Brief Description: _____
_____
_____

- Country of Origin: _____
- Extraction Method: _____
- Plant Parts: _____
- Botanical Family: _____
- Chemical Families: _____
- Aroma: _____
- Note: _____

PRECAUTIONS _____

Therapeutic Properties

USES

Bones/Joints: _____

_____

Circulatory: _____

_____

Digestive: _____

_____

Immune: _____

_____

Lymphatic: _____

_____

Mental/Emotional: _____

_____

Muscular/Joint: _____

_____

Reproductive: _____

_____

Respiratory: _____

_____

Skin: _____

_____

Urinary: _____

_____

SAFETY

_____

_____

_____

ESSENTIAL OIL DATASHEET FORM

Use this form to create your own datasheets for essential oils you have in your collection. You will need to do some research online or from books on hand to gather the information regarding your particular oil.

Oil Name: _____

Brief Description: _____
_____
_____

- Country of Origin: _____
- Extraction Method: _____
- Plant Parts: _____
- Botanical Family: _____
- Chemical Families: _____
- Aroma: _____
- Note: _____

PRECAUTIONS _____

Therapeutic Properties

USES

Bones/Joints: _____
_____

Circulatory: _____
_____

Digestive: _____
_____

Immune: _____
_____

Lymphatic: _____
_____

Mental/Emotional: _____
_____

Muscular/Joint: _____
_____

Reproductive: _____
_____

Respiratory: _____
_____

Skin: _____
_____

Urinary: _____
_____

SAFETY

_____
_____
_____

ESSENTIAL OIL DATASHEET FORM

Use this form to create your own datasheets for essential oils you have in your collection. You will need to do some research online or from books on hand to gather the information regarding your particular oil.

Oil Name: _____

Brief Description: _____
_____
_____

- **Country of Origin:** _____
- **Extraction Method:** _____
- **Plant Parts:** _____
- **Botanical Family:** _____
- **Chemical Families:** _____
- **Aroma:** _____
- **Note:** _____

PRECAUTIONS _____

Therapeutic Properties

USES

Bones/Joints: _____
_____

Circulatory: _____
_____

Digestive: _____
_____

Immune: _____
_____

Lymphatic: _____
_____

Mental/Emotional: _____
_____

Muscular/Joint: _____
_____

Reproductive: _____
_____

Respiratory: _____
_____

Skin: _____
_____

Urinary: _____
_____

SAFETY

_____
_____
_____

ESSENTIAL OIL DATASHEET FORM

Use this form to create your own datasheets for essential oils you have in your collection. You will need to do some research online or from books on hand to gather the information regarding your particular oil.

Oil Name: _____

Brief Description: _____
_____
_____

- Country of Origin: _____
- Extraction Method: _____
- Plant Parts: _____
- Botanical Family: _____
- Chemical Families: _____
- Aroma: _____
- Note: _____

PRECAUTIONS _____

Therapeutic Properties

USES

Bones/Joints: _____
_____

Circulatory: _____
_____

Digestive: _____
_____

Immune: _____
_____

Lymphatic: _____
_____

Mental/Emotional: _____
_____

Muscular/Joint: _____
_____

Reproductive: _____
_____

Respiratory: _____
_____

Skin: _____
_____

Urinary: _____
_____

SAFETY

_____
_____
_____

ESSENTIAL OIL DATASHEET FORM

Use this form to create your own datasheets for essential oils you have in your collection. You will need to do some research online or from books on hand to gather the information regarding your particular oil.

Oil Name: _____

Brief Description: _____
_____
_____

- Country of Origin: _____
- Extraction Method: _____
- Plant Parts: _____
- Botanical Family: _____
- Chemical Families: _____
- Aroma: _____
- Note: _____

PRECAUTIONS _____

Therapeutic Properties

USES

Bones/Joints: _____
_____

Circulatory: _____
_____

Digestive: _____
_____

Immune: _____
_____

Lymphatic: _____
_____

Mental/Emotional: _____
_____

Muscular/Joint: _____
_____

Reproductive: _____
_____

Respiratory: _____
_____

Skin: _____
_____

Urinary: _____
_____

SAFETY

_____
_____
_____

ESSENTIAL OIL DATASHEET FORM

Use this form to create your own datasheets for essential oils you have in your collection. You will need to do some research online or from books on hand to gather the information regarding your particular oil.

Oil Name: _____

Brief Description: _____
_____
_____

- Country of Origin: _____
- Extraction Method: _____
- Plant Parts: _____
- Botanical Family: _____
- Chemical Families: _____
- Aroma: _____
- Note: _____

PRECAUTIONS _____

Therapeutic Properties

239

USES

Bones/Joints: _____
_____

Circulatory: _____
_____

Digestive: _____
_____

Immune: _____
_____

Lymphatic: _____
_____

Mental/Emotional: _____
_____

Muscular/Joint: _____
_____

Reproductive: _____
_____

Respiratory: _____
_____

Skin: _____
_____

Urinary: _____
_____

SAFETY

_____
_____
_____

ESSENTIAL OIL DATASHEET FORM

Use this form to create your own datasheets for essential oils you have in your collection. You will need to do some research online or from books on hand to gather the information regarding your particular oil.

Oil Name: _____

Brief Description: _____
_____
_____

- Country of Origin: _____
- Extraction Method: _____
- Plant Parts: _____
- Botanical Family: _____
- Chemical Families: _____
- Aroma: _____
- Note: _____

PRECAUTIONS _____

Therapeutic Properties

USES

Bones/Joints: _____
_____

Circulatory: _____
_____

Digestive: _____
_____

Immune: _____
_____

Lymphatic: _____
_____

Mental/Emotional: _____
_____

Muscular/Joint: _____
_____

Reproductive: _____
_____

Respiratory: _____
_____

Skin: _____
_____

Urinary: _____
_____

SAFETY

_____
_____
_____

ESSENTIAL OIL DATASHEET FORM

Use this form to create your own datasheets for essential oils you have in your collection. You will need to do some research online or from books on hand to gather the information regarding your particular oil.

Oil Name: ☐

Brief Description: _____
_____
_____

- Country of Origin: _____
- Extraction Method: _____
- Plant Parts: _____
- Botanical Family: _____
- Chemical Families: _____
- Aroma: _____
- Note: _____

PRECAUTIONS _____

Therapeutic Properties

USES

Bones/Joints: _____
_____

Circulatory: _____
_____

Digestive: _____
_____

Immune: _____
_____

Lymphatic: _____
_____

Mental/Emotional: _____
_____

Muscular/Joint: _____
_____

Reproductive: _____
_____

Respiratory: _____
_____

Skin: _____
_____

Urinary: _____
_____

SAFETY

_____
_____
_____